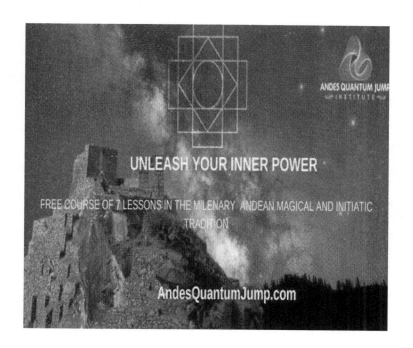

Design and layout of the Book:

Tomas Gomez

Edited by:

Tom Wagner, Donna Osborn

First Edition:

April 2019

For more information, on the content of this book, training and seminars in the USA on the Andean Tradition, as taught in the book, visit our web site:

www.andesquantumjump.com

You may send us a message to:

rodfuentes @andesquantumjump.com

Or follow us in our social media

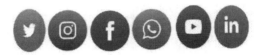

Dr. Rod Fuentes

"Andes Quantum Jump Institute"

.

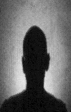

"Your Aura, Personal Atmosphere or Energy Bubble"
(Subconscious Mind)

FREE COURSE OF 4 LESSONS ON THIS FIELD OF SUBTLE ENERGIES COMPOSED OF
THOUGHTS AND DESIRES THAT MATERIALIZE OUR LIFE AND EVERYTHING

AndesQuantumJump.com

ACKNOWLEDGMENTS

My acknowledgments to master healer, and Paqo, Don Joaquín Freire, who instructed me on the principles of the "Guardians of Wisdom" in the Andes Mountains of Chile. He showed me the 4 worlds of reality, the 4 levels of perception or "ñawis," the Andean Codes and the 7 sacred Rites of the Mountains. He also explained the Sacred secrets of ancient wisdom of the Andes Mountains where I was born, grew and still live today. He dispelled from my mind many errors that I had acquired concerning the true spiritual path.

I also want to thank the other "Guardians of Wisdom" who, like him, kept alive the flame of knowledge in the Andean mountains; but especially to the great teacher R.V.N who took me as his disciple and instructed me in the true "spirituality" and in the principles of the 49 Lessons of "Andean Illumination." These teachings guided me at an early age from my personal visions to rediscover the ancestral, timeless and transcendental wisdom of the sacred lands of the Andes, where I had the privilege of being born. A place where, from time immemorial, spiritual giants walked.

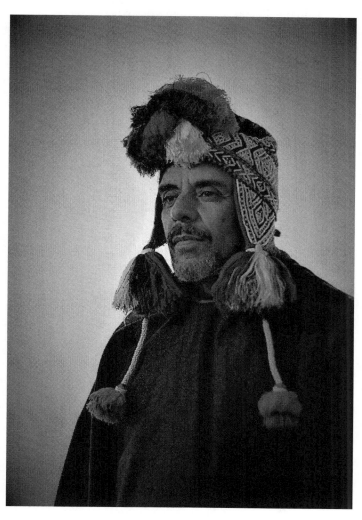

Dr. Fuentes in the sacred Andean vestments.

FOREWARD

Have you ever wondered what wisdom, secrets and technologies have been lost by mankind? No matter how far we advance in technology, as a group mind, we feel that we have lost something long ago. We left a treasure of information in the past, as we rejected the old superstitions, and now embrace pure material science. What was contained in the Library of Alexandria? How were the pyramids built? Did the ancients have a better relationship with the supernatural and divinity, than we do now, within our religious institutions? The desire to know our past and recover what was lost long ago is manifested within all cultures. The quest for the past and its secrets drives us into the realms of imaginations and preposterous theories because our material egos will not accept a response of, "I don't know the answer to that question." False pride produced by egotistical intellectuals who refuse to accept that the ancients were smarter than them, block all new ideas about our ancient heritage. When we cannot explain something, we then create a source or power without facts to support our beliefs. Unfortunately, we bring religious and cultural bias into our theories that block intellectuals from pursuing any real knowledge from the distant past. But what if there was a time capsule from centuries ago that was found that contained the wisdom of the ancient people? Even better, what if it contained living knowledge instead of art works or almost undecipherable writings. Wouldn't it be great to talk to these ancient people, like the Incas, and ask them to share their wisdom with us? Dr. Rod Fuentes has been trained by the descendants of these ancient Inca Priests, early in his childhood, and has presented this book containing their philosophies.

We marvel at the technologies used to build their temples and infrastructures with primitive tools. Where did they get this technology and why hasn't it been passed down to us? Lay people and amateur archeologists have a different opinion than the mainstream anthropologists. The later believe in pure science and will not accept any pseudo-science, nor will they accept that the ancients had contact with extra-terrestrial civilizations that shared their technologies with them. The former believe that they were using magical, occult or mystical forces to create their civilization. The traditional mainstream scientific groups defend their analysis of these civilizations by just admitting that they have not discovered all the answers yet, but in time, a practical and natural answer will reveal itself.

Dr. Fuentes explains how the Inca Culture had a strong relationship with all nature, and not just the physical form. They had a secret knowledge of the spiritual qualities of every aspect of nature and could communicate with the spiritual guardians of plants, rocks, rivers, storms and all life. To modern man this might appear to be nothing but pagan superstitions, but how did they survive for nearly 500 years isolated in such a harsh and dangerous environment? Under your present conditions, do you think that your knowledge is sufficient enough to not only survive, but to prosper, so your children and grandchildren could prosper also? What did these Inca priest know that gave them the ability to live in these conditions? We know they had a culture and religion that was over 10,000 years old, that bound them together in unity. Their culture and religion must have come with them from their place of origins, possibly from Siberia, or perhaps the legendary island of Lemuria. Yes, the Incas have a legend that their first king came from a sunken island in the Pacific Ocean.

Only recently has more information come to light that might give this legend some credibility. In 1936, Edgar Cayce, the great American Sleeping Prophet, mentioned that there was a great island in the Pacific Ocean with an advance civilization that had colonized Asia and the Pacific coasts of South America before sinking into the sea. The Oceanic Institute announced that they have discovered a possible land bridge that existed in the past between Peru and the Archipelago Islands before sinking into the sea. In New Zealand, which was believed to have only been occupied by humans around 850 A.D., a wall has been found that looks very similar to the techniques used by the Incas. They have also discovered a large sunken land mass near New Zealand that could have been a lost continent before being submerged under the sea. This new discovery, although needing more research to confirm its validity, gives more credibility to the legends of Mu (Lemuria) and the origins of the civilizations in South America. With the recent discovery of a lost Inca village living isolated from the world in the mid Twentieth Century, we now can look into the past to not only understand the Incas, but the legend of the people of Lemuria (Mu), Madame Blavatsky, in her book "The Secret

Doctrine," mentions the legends of the Lemurian people many times as a fact. It is only a matter of time before mainstream historians and researchers will be able to present their theories as fact.

Dr. Rod Fuentes has given us an insight into how ancient cultures lived, thought and practiced their philosophies of life by revealing the secrets of the Inca Priesthood's Code of the Andes.   After numerous conversations with Dr. Fuentes, I believe his book fully explains these codes through modern examples and languages that we can understand and apply in our lives. This is not a concise history of the Inca people, to be read for personal enjoyment, but a philosophy that all people, religions, faiths and governments could use to benefit themselves and others.   It does not contradict anyone's personal faith, but rather improves upon it.   It is not a new religion or governmental concept, nor does it focus on any new age construct, or beliefs. However, it can benefit all people and strengthen their personal lives with practical Exercises introduced throughout this book.

As stated previously, Dr. Fuentes began his training as an Inca Priest at the age of 14 years. His desire to help people, led him into the medical field, the ministry, motivational coaching and into the field of Hypno-therapy. He is dedicated to the Andean Code of Anyi, which is the Code of sacred reciprocity, which expresses itself in service to others. Dr. Rod Fuentes is a holistic healer and treats all levels of the human being. He does not just look at the physical body, but also the mind and the spirit of an individual. He not only tries to help people by pointing out errors in their thinking or how they should live and treat others, but he goes deeper into the areas of the soul. He believes if the soul and the mind are sick, then it will eventually express itself in the body and in the mind. He has revealed in this book many of the problems, and cures, for people living in our stressful modern life.

The Inca priests have come down out of the mountains to help us in these troubling times. They have given their Codes for us to use for our benefit. At a very young age, Dr. Fuentes met one of these priests while hiking in the Andes Mountains, and received their training. He also has immersed himself in Western sciences to become an exceptional teacher and spiritual guide. He has studied and practiced these Codes his entire life and helped many people. I was blessed to have been introduced to him in the 1990's and since the day I met him, I have called him a friend, teacher and spiritual guide.

In conclusion, the Inca Priests have declared that the prophecy of the Pachacuti, which is the return of the Golden Man, will follow the time when the Condor (Andean people) flies with the Eagle (the people of North America). Hardships and calamites have been prophesized to come upon us, and our modern technologies can't prevent it, but the Incas have given us a philosophy that can help us endure all hardships. They survived a holocaust and extreme environmental hardships for centuries and have proven that their Codes of Life work. In the spirit of Ayni, they wish to share their blessings with the world. Dr. Rod Fuentes is a bridge, between South America and North America and teaches that the two hemispheres must come together to survive. We all would benefit greatly from his book as he reveals the teachings of the Andean Codes of Life.

Dennis Osborn

Andes Quantum Jump Institute,

Memphis, Tennessee, U.S.A.

This page left blank

INTRODUCTION

We are on the verge of one of the most critical moments in the history of the Earth. The last decades were the decades of "more," in which society tried to buy happiness through the acquisition of more "things," but research has shown that since the 1950s we are more depressed, more violent, more suicidal and more stressed than ever. Materialism offered apparent salvation, but more and more people began to realize that more "things" cannot buy more happiness and there is a very small relationship between the two.

The last decades have also been of an extraordinary and unimaginable technological development, but gigantic problems have also emerged, which puts us today amid changes and threats totally unthinkable for the generations of the past. Unstable global economy and politics, advancing artificial intelligence, controversies of climate change with the melting of glaciers, the extinction of species, chemical pollution, destruction of marine plankton, natural disasters of cataclysmic proportions and the growing chronic diseases which have occurred and continue to occur, locate us in one of the most difficult recorded stages for mankind.

All this is in complete contradiction to the happy, prosperous and harmonious life that we all hoped it would be to live in the New Millennium. Likewise, many of the promises made by science, governments, the pharmaceutical industry and large companies have not been able to bring peace, prosperity, health or happiness on the planet. A time has come when we need to look elsewhere for the resources to face the challenges of the 21st century that are unparalleled in the recorded history of humanity.

The possibilities are simple and clear, either we take a quantum leap towards a new level of life, or we descend deeper into chaos and despair, perhaps on the path to complete annihilation of the human species. Although we still depend on technology and suppliers of goods and services, the need is greater than ever to take responsibility for our own thoughts, feelings, behaviors and beliefs. If we succeed, we could make a massive leap in our own evolution. The decisions we make now and the actions we take will affect the future, not only for us, but for our descendants.

Imagine for a moment that someone takes you to a library hidden in the highest mountains, inaccessible to the world, containing a book of wisdom that contained the Codes of the highest importance to humanity. These Codes instructed the Qeros, the Incan Priesthood, to survive in the harshest of environments, with lack of food or heat. This remnant endured the most atrocious genocide in the history of the Inca Nation.

I refer to the four levels of reality and their perception and the "Andean Codes" that the old "Guardians of Wisdom," the Q'eros in the Andean mountains, kept intact for the arrival of these times. Among them, the Andean Code which is the most important of all is, AYNI, or "Sacred Reciprocity" with all things and with all human beings, which, if humanity incorporated it, we would instantaneously behold a heaven on Earth without delay.

Without adhering to this single Code, which offers the most positive and valuable forces in your life, which includes positive thinking, personal achievements, prosperity, health and many other good things that the teachings of this book impart, one runs the risk of becoming corrupted, negative and harmful to oneself as well as to others. In such cases the "soul" of the individual's behavior, and the intentions, will always be selfish and harmful.

The adherence to this knowledge that involves the "Andean Codes" has allowed the Q'eros to live more than 12,000 feet above sea level with no police force, no judges, no jails, no hospitals and there is no crime between them, nor orphans, nor abandoned children, nor broken families. They have been cured of their diseases, far from any hospital and with a great lack of food. They have had strong and healthy teeth without dentists. Inside their stone houses, they have survived temperatures below 14 degrees Fahrenheit. These examples seem impossible or unthinkable for our modern Western "reality platforms," or "models of the world."

Without civil or criminal law, they live exclusively under the "model of the world" contained in these Andean Codes that ancient Incan wisdom bequeathed to them. For centuries they have had inner spiritual experiences and are an example of survival under the most extreme conditions. And they gave to us these wonderful Codes to teach in this New Era and these new times to the whole world.

Where is the enormous power of such codes that the Q'eros fully demonstrated? The power of such "Andean Codes" is in the fundamental teaching, contained intrinsically in them, that says that the problems we face must be resolved at the level of reality in which they were created; generally, in a level higher than that in which they were manifested. Because if we try to correct the problem only at the level that it manifested, there will be a temporary solution, or none at all. We can add to this, that all the problems and situations we face are solved, without exception, from the highest level of reality, as I will show, and I will teach to you in this book.

Is this something that you would be interested to know? If so, keep reading ...

PREAMBLE

The Andean Codes are seven very ancient Quechua words, the language of the Andes, that are stamped on the earth and on our planet everywhere; they are the key to everything.

We encounter these Codes through our feelings for the stones, the plants, the trees and the whole of nature. These Codes are living truths that are observed in a mountain, in the rivers, in the winds, in the clouds, in the animals and in the human beings. The Codes are the spirit of life and the realization of everything.

The Andean Codes are also what allows you to enter the inner world and go through the door that communicates with the essence of reality and Pachamama, the Mother of all.

Table of Contents

*In this introductory book, we will be using the Quechua Language throughout. The repetition of words and phrases is intentional and for emphasis. The Quechua language was not written and was based on phonetics and a dialect chain which results in different spellings according to the author.

*This book contains extensive exercises to develop the higher levels of reality from where change can be obtained but should not be construed as medical advice. The suggestions and exercises contained herein should NOT take the place of your medical doctor's guidance.

CHAPTER ONE

Ayahuasca as a "master plant"

Many people are hoping to reach the state of illumination[1] or spiritual development and enlightenment by the use of herbs, or "master plants," such as Ayahuasca. It is this belief about this herb, which has become extremely well known and famous all over the world, even in countries far away from the Andes such as Europe and the United States of America, that I need to speak truthfully about its powers and effects. Thousands of people with good intentions, but possessing a false idea, goal or hope, arrive at Cuzco or the Amazon Jungle of Peru daily, to ingest this herb. A small fortune is spent hoping that an herb will be a cure for every disease, or addiction, and will also grant enlightenment.

There is a great misrepresentation of how things really are, and the greatest Guardians of Wisdom in the Andes Mountains, where I have lived all my life, like master Don Joaquin Freire, were fully aware of this mistake. From the very

---

[1] Illumination: from the Latin, "to throw light into."

beginning of my spiritual journey, when I consulted him about these plants, he warned me about this problem.

The herbs and plants that the local shamans use, which are native to the South American jungles, are considered "sacred plants," or "master plants," and must always be treated with great respect by those who consume them as a medicine. But never for a moment should anyone consider them as a shortcut to heaven, nor as a recreational "drug." None of these beliefs have anything to do with the real and very useful purposes that these sacred plants contain, having been given to us by the Great Mother of Nature.

By invoking the name of Ayahuasca, I include here a short dissertation about the "Master Plant." I wish to inform those that have this same disillusionment that I had. In order to spare the many a lot of fruitless efforts, sacrifices and expenses that otherwise could lead them to loss, frustration and unnecessary dangers, I wish to dispel this error from their minds. The partaking of Ayahuasca is only recommended by the Guardians of Wisdom as a support for psychological treatments in the cases of addictions, alcoholism, very intense depression, or psychosomatic illnesses. It is a valuable and extraordinary tool for all these cases when under the guidance of an expert. In many of these cases, there have been good results achieved for the patient, but there have also been failures that people ignore.

What Ayahuasca really does is take a person consuming the herb to an experience very similar to physical death. Perhaps this is the reason why it came to be confused in the minds of millions, with an herb that causes "illumination or spiritual Enlightenment," because after the death experience, there comes a rebirth and a renewal; but that has never been the case with Ayahuasca.

Those who know and live in the Andes, know that Ayahuasca is a good remedy for some mental illnesses under the care of an expert healer. The ingestion of Ayahuasca causes a very difficult and strong reaction, which is often a painful and agonizing experience, that must be carefully watched by an expert. Those who consume it, observe memories passing in front of their mental eyes; these memories are very vivid and remarkable events of their lives, associated with their problems and troubles, just as it happens in a near death experience.

What really occurs, is the accessing of the unconscious data base, with all its content of past experiences, by use of the plant, which is similar to a near death experience.

In most cases, Ayahuasca also causes a series of rather unpleasant physical symptoms, such as vomiting and diarrhea. Because it is a true purge of traumas from the past, these are seen vividly and dramatically with eyes of the mind; and because it also causes the release of stagnant energies and trapped emotions in the person, your body and your mind are affected. It forces one to deal with everything that is at the root of their problems and troubles, such as addictions, alcoholism, depression, or psychosomatic illnesses.

The author of this book personally treats many cases of addictions, depression, and alcoholism, with hypnotherapy and NLP (Neuro Linguistic Programing). I have recommended the use of Ayahuasca to some of my patients, under the care of an expert, in those situations when they are of a very severe nature.

Ayni – Andean Gratitude

To those who thought that Ayahuasca would lead them to illumination, I write these words in kindness.　Don Joaquin Freire, one of the Guardians of Wisdom in the Andes Mountains, spoke to me many years ago, when I asked him about the possibility of illumination; because at an early age I had the same beliefs about this herb's powers. He told me to stop thinking about this false belief that Ayahuasca has the ability to cause illumination. He said that I should refer to what all the true masters of wisdom in the Andes have done, that I should embrace AYNI, instead of an immediate path to Heaven. He said that to reach the highest levels of consciousness that I should embrace the Sacred Reciprocity of the "energies of the Universe," as all true Guardians of Wisdom have done, for untold centuries. He taught me that only AYNI (Andean Gratitude) would guide people to real "illumination and spiritual enlightenment" and to the different degrees of consciousness in the human experience; this is something that all Guardians of Wisdom always aim to accomplish. But this is something that can never be achieved by an herb, regardless of how powerful as a mental medicine it could be.

In short, this is the same message I received in the beginning of my spiritual training from a great Paquos of the Andes. As stated, I also thought that Ayahuasca would grant me illumination and higher levels of consciousness, when the truth is, only <u>Ayni</u> can give you enlightenment.

In this book is the path that I teach to others today. Dispelling one of the most frequent mistakes in the minds of those who look toward the ancient Andean sacred tradition for spiritual development and enlightenment, I repeat a second time, if you really want to obtain true "spiritual" results, and you have been using Ayahuasca, believing that this "master plant" or herb could help you reach that goal, you already know the mistakes of that false belief. *Correct your false beliefs now* and move away from Ayahuasca and embrace Ayni; there you will find what you have been looking for all along. This will help you acquire your desired spiritual goals.

.

CHAPTER TWO

Understanding the Andean Codes

The understanding and application of Ayni and the other six ancient Codes, gives us a new and improved vision of life and the world. They make up a true successful operating system when it is set in motion within a society or community, as was the case with the Qeros. Individually, as a spiritual discipline for the individual who practices alone, they contain the essence of knowledge that moves the universe. By understanding these Codes, and applying them, we access a different vision, which will be a powerful engine for change and fulfillment.

It is a worldview in which the interest is not placed on how the universe works, but on how one has to align oneself to the universe and live it 'in the everyday.' In order to apply the Codes correctly and fully, perceptions of life must be developed from one of the higher levels of reality, which will be explained in Chapter Five and thereafter.

Introduction to the Andean Codes

The *"Andean Codes"* are the philosophical and ideological system of the Society of the Guardians of the Wisdom, or Paqos. Nobody knows when they were grasped by the mind and soul of the ancient people and highest initiates and priests in the Andes. But what we know for sure is that the inhabitants of the Qero nation made a very practical and daily use of them.

As stated in the Introduction of this book, they lived at over 12,000 feet above sea level. They have never had a police force, nor judges, nor jails, nor hospitals. There has never been crime among them, neither orphans nor abandoned children, nor broken families. They have lived without civil or criminal law and with only the Codes. They have always healed themselves from their illnesses, away from any hospital, and with a big scarcity of food. They have had strong, healthy teeth without ever going to the dentist. They survive at temperatures below 10 degrees Celsius inside their stone abodes, something that is impossible or unthinkable for our modern western "reality platforms" or "models of the world."

They have lived exclusively and solely under the magical and initiatic "model of the world" that the Inca priests bequeathed upon them from past centuries. They have had mystical experiences while surviving under the most extreme conditions. Based on these seven "Andean Codes," they adhere tightly to these paradigms of the initiatic and magical society from which they descended.

As one of the Qeros explained to me, this "model of a magical world" is made up of these seven fundamental principles which created for them a true "Operational System of Group Consciousness" or "Integrative Operational System of Society" (SOIS) which has enabled them to achieve the above mentioned conditions.

The symbols, which have been kept alive in Peru and Chile for several hundreds of years representing this millenary initiatic wisdom of the "Codes," are somehow similar to others found in European and American Hermeticism groups from the Seventeenth to the Twentieth Centuries. These are the symbols of polarity, the three forces and the tawantin, "quaternary" or evolutionary triad.

If anybody takes on the task of raising his/her perception to those levels of reality, these principles are very practical and completely applicable to everyday life. When following them *individually*, one by one, they allow us to live a completely fulfilled life. And when applying them *collectively* they allow us to replicate a healthy and happy society without crime, without police force, without judges, without evils upon society.

The 7 "Andean Codes" are important referents which make it possible for life to be easier, more dignified and completely aligned and interconnected with universal Forces and energies that a allow us a world vision which is essentially *practical* and applicable.

The "guardian of the wisdom" of the Andes are not so much interested in knowing how the Universe works but in *how to act in order to align with the Universe*, therefore, everything they learn and teach is direct and applied to daily life.

Here below you find the 7 codes
and how these codes are organized:

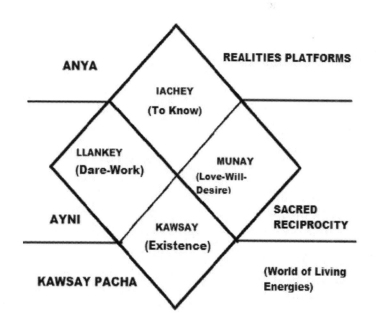

7 Andean Codes

KAWSAY
(Existence)

- Everything that exists is alive and is living energy.
- That universal energy (Kawsay) gives existence to everything.
- Everything we see, even when it seems inert – a glass, a stone – is alive because of that energy.
- The energy of objects, of everything that exists, is affected by our thought and intention; we can thus program and deprogram this energy.
- This influence is greater when I put my MUNAY into action (another Andean Code that is a combination of three forces: Will -Love– Desire – mixed into one divine force for good.)
- The energy is always fluid and healthy in all things, except for human beings who, by their negative thoughts and emotions, can stagnate, coagulate, and transform it into poisonous and harmful energy called HUCHA.
- Person and object are one thing, what is inside is like what is outside. The external world is a reflection of our internal world.
- So, all things concerning our life – good or bad – exist because we have given them existence

(Kawsay). Because we we were created as creators of our realities

- Likewise, the things that do not exist in our life – good or bad – do not exist because we have not given them existence.
- I can, through my intention, give existence to what I want and remove existence from the things I do not want in my life.
- I can consciously affect the existence and energy of things in my life through speech and movement; this will have a powerful impact on this energy of existence (Kawsay.)

LLANKAY
(pronounced Yankay)
To Dare, To Work
Through work and being bold you attain.

MUNAY
Love- Will- Desire
This mixture is a magical power that makes anything possible.

IACHEY
(pronounce Iachay)
To Know; Wisdom

You may get wisdom and materialize all your experiences in symbols that allows you to avoid repeating again what is not necessary.

ANYA
Reality Platforms

Learn to understand that there are many different models of the world and that you may live in one or many of them. Your results in life will be according to the Reality Platform on which you seek to exist and has nothing to do with your skills or capacities. You will learn to respect and accept different points of view because you understand they are just different viewpoints of the truth. These wisdom programs sprouted from a collective mind that lived on the highest levels of perception and consciousness and were bequeathed by them, the Paqos (Priests) to the New Era.

AYNI
Sacred Reciprocity

The first Principle taught by God to mankind is the interchange, the "Sacred Reciprocity," of the Energies of the Universe in everything, everywhere and with everyone.

It is the first principle taught by the Andean Paqos. The concept of <u>Ayni</u>, or "Sacred Reciprocity of the Energies," means a completely disinterested altruistic exchange of energies, physical and non-physical, among all beings in the Universe. It is something that all beings, celestial and terrestrial, naturally and constantly do, except for mankind. Mankind is the only exceptional species in the whole Universe, both visible and invisible worlds, created and offered free will to practice Ayni, or to abstain. Ayni says "give always something **before** asking." It involves helping a friend in need by offering help or at least offering a prayer; it is a "Sacred Compensation." Ayni is "spiritual" reciprocity that extends beyond the immediate return, although, by definition, it guarantees a return, so you often receive more than what was given. What you receive back in return often includes energies in love, health, protection, money, knowledge and other material and spiritual things as well. Sacred Reciprocity (Ayni), in its fundamental spirit, is like the evolutionary force of the natural world and the energetic law of the cosmos, which includes the material world and beyond the physical into the spiritual realms. It is said that Sacred Reciprocity (Ayni) was the first principle that God, or the Creator, made known to human beings when men were nearer to the "gods," just after their creation, which was necessary for their complete well-being.

KAWSAY PACHA
World of Living Energies

Learn to live at all times in the world of "existence" or "living energies" through the principle of (Kawsay) and the Sacred Reciprocity (AYNI) thus making your life something incredible beyond belief.

Andean Gratitude

Huiracocha, or God the Creator, spoke "AYNI INAIKUCH ES," that, in Qechua language, the language of the Andes, means: "Live in Ayni." The Ayni is one of the most important secrets of the Andean Codes and also a cardinal principle in the teaching of the "Guardians of Wisdom." It must be expressed not only in acts, but also in good thoughts and feelings towards each other. It also expresses itself in other energies, as taught in different places and chapters of this book. Ayni is a real treasure for all humankind, but it is something completely unknown and ignored for the most part of the human race, which causes much suffering for mankind by not following this Divine Decree.

Kindness, good feelings, and goodwill towards others, are all equally powerful expressions of some form of Ayni, but that's only the beginning. Ayni not only creates positive events, such as happy situations in our lives, including prosperity, health, love, and anything desired, but also spiritual illumination and spiritual advancement. Ayni also imprints favorable energy codes in our aura, or "sphere of luminous energy," that will result in innumerable other benefits, too, which is something that could never be imagined or even expected from the "master plant" called "Ayahuasca," regardless of how powerful it may be in the curing of different diseases of mankind.   After you have absorbed the Andean Code Ayni, and become familiar with the different reality platforms, there will be some final words on Ayahuasca towards the end of this book. All this will be fully explained as you continue to read.

CHAPTER THREE

The Mythical "Guardians of Wisdom" In the Andean Mountains Fulfillment of Prophecy

In 1949, in the sacred Mountains of the Andes, there was a terrible earthquake under a monastery near Cuzco, Peru, which divided the land and brought to light an ancient Incan temple of gold. That was the signal that the prophecies of the "time to come" had begun. The prophecy of the "Guardians of Wisdom" said that this time in which we live is the moment of the "great encounter" called "mastay;" that is, the reintegration of the peoples of the four cardinal points in the world. Once considered a kind of myth, in the early 1990s, the Q'eros people came down from the Mountains to fulfill this prophecy with the "Andean Codes," and to share their ancient tradition of wisdom and healing medicine with the needy and desperate modern world.

History

In one of the most difficult recorded stages of human history, the Q'eros responded to the call of the ancient prophecies for the "reintegration," with the aim of guiding us on the journey of returning, once again, to spirituality. Composed of seven villages with more than 600 families, together they were called the Q`ero Nation. They were revealed to the modern world in 1955. Remarkably, they kept intact the "Andean Codes," that they offered as a new paradigm for humanity, among which is the Andean Code AYNI, or "Sacred Reciprocity," one of the most valuable Codes that they possess and practice.

The first expedition high up into the Andes mountains, to the "guardians of knowledge," was directed by Oscar Nuñez del Prado. His goal was to find a people that, according to myth and legend, had moved to the highest mountains when the Spanish conquistadores invaded Peru in 1532. In one of the most terrible genocides humanity has ever known, the invading conquistadores almost completely destroyed the Incan Empire. The Q'ero were considered the last Incas and kept hidden, in the unattainable heights of the mountains, the ancient traditions that existed in the Andes of Peru, Ecuador and Chile.

Prophecy of World Harmony and Order

For nearly 500 years, the "guardians of knowledge", or Paqos of the Q'ero Nation, passed between them a prophecy about a great change, in which the world would turn around, and in which "harmony and order" would be restored, by putting an end to chaos and disorder. Through the ancient teachings of the priests, teachers and guardians of the wisdom, the Seven Andean Codes can completely change the world by being well applied to modern life.

When Oscar Nuñez del Prado's team approached the Q'eros' villages, they were greeted by the men of the village. The women and children were hidden because they thought that the Spaniards had finally found them. When Oscar Nuñez del Prado asked the men who they were, the men replied that "we are the children of the Sun; our father is the Sun and our mother is the Earth (Pachamama in the Quechua language of the Q'eros)."

Oscar Nuñez del Prado saw that the Q'eros preserved and practiced the traditional ceremonies and the spiritual teachings of the "Guardians of Wisdom." These ageless teachings survived the genocide carried out by the Spaniards almost 500 years prior and were exactly like the myths of the extinct Incas. It turned out that the Q'eros were the people Oscar was looking for, being one of the Inca groups who fled to the mountains when their Empire was destroyed by the Conquistadores.

The Incas knew that their 10,000-year-old Andean spiritual tradition and prophesy were in grave danger. Since the time of their genocide, for nearly 500 years, they had watched and administered the teachings of the "Andean Codes" that had been taught in the Andes for thousands of years. The Q'eros knew that their contact with the ancient wisdom should not be forgotten or lost.

The conquerors had searched for gold in the Q'ero villages relentlessly, but were unsuccessful, because of the wisdom and knowledge of the Q'ero priests and priestesses. They simply kept the conquerors away by using their strong connection with the powers of Earth and mountains and their handling of the "living energies" that they called "Existence." When summoned by the Priests, the forces of nature responded. The trail of the conquerors was blocked by nature itself, through the rivers of drowning water, and the rocks of the mountains that fell on them.

Dr. Rod Fuentes with Juan Nuñez del Prado,
Oscar del Prado's son

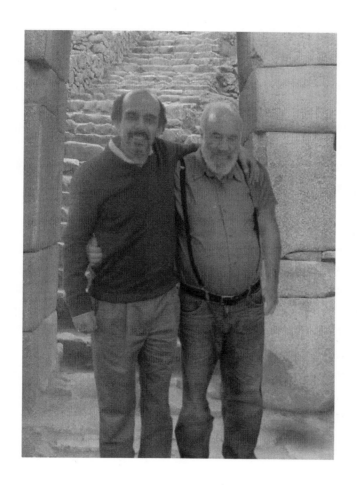

In 1532, when the conquerors seized the land and brought the Christian faith of Europe, the Inca Empire and its 10,000-year-old traditions were slowly forgotten, and the Inca priests who fled, became a myth of a people that disappeared in the legendary snowy mountains of the Andes. From that time, the Q'eros were completely isolated for almost 500 years. Their ancient wisdom was very pure and not affected by any other culture, teachings or religions. Their wisdom, called the Andean Codes, was transmitted verbally from mouth to ear, from father and mother, to son and daughter, for many generations.

In 1959, the Q'eros, being fully aware that the conquerors were no longer in the Andes, re-appeared during the celebration of the "Return of the Pleiades." The participating South American pilgrims were surprised, and the crowd parted to let the Q'ero priest, who carried the Inca emblem of the Sun, make his way to the top of the mountain to announce that the time of the prophecies was near.

In the early 1990s, the Q'ero people saw signs on the horizon and realized that it was time for the "Guardians of Wisdom" to reveal themselves. These Guardians descended from the mountains with their colorful clothes of the rainbow and spoke prophecies about a new era in which great changes would begin to happen on the planet. They prophesied:

"When there is a tear in the sky that makes the sunshine and harm us, when the glaciers melt, when the weather changes and natural disasters arise and when the Condor is about to disappear, we must walk and share our tradition and wisdom with the world."

According to this prophecy, it is time for the people of the West to wake up from a deep sleep and reach their human potential, applying these Codes to their life; because a new era has already been born, and the modern human being of intellect and brain is now being touched by the heart and soul of the Andes. These "Guardians of Wisdom," or Paqos, extended widely and openly their traditions; traditions which survived from before the Spanish conquest, a time when the Incan Empire was spread from southern Colombia to southern Chile. They teach that by walking with deep spiritual awareness and presence, you can read how the living energy of the Universe (Kausay) is reflected in your own soul; then you can change and control this living energy within yourself and affect your own reality and that of other people and the external world in general.

The natives of the ancient Inca traditions or "Guardians of Wisdom," who should not be confused with the shamans, call themselves "Paqos," which means "reborn," and also Andean priest or priestess, or "Initiate of the Andean mountains." They are also known as "masters of living energy," or "guardians of knowledge," and believe that the journey to unite with our highest potential occurs from a place of deep self-knowledge and from the inner power of the brain and soul within us; never from substances outside of our being.

Finally, the Paqos, in the early 1990s, descended to offer their ancient teachings to the West, to the fulfillment of prophecy, in preparation for the day when the Northern Eagle and Southern Condor (the Americas) fly together again. These descendants of the Incas of ancient times believe that sacred reciprocity (Ayni), love and compassion, will be the force that will guide this great union of peoples and traditions. This future spoken of by the "guardians of knowledge" must now come from the West, because they are the ones that have caused the greatest damage to Mother Earth. This will be done through the application of the 7 Andean Codes. For this reason, Westerners have the moral responsibility to rebuild a harmonious relationship with nature again, and with Mother Earth and Pachamama.

This ancient prophecy states that the United States will provide the physical strength, or the body; Europe will provide the mental aspect or wisdom; and the heart (or Love) will be provided by South America.

The author of this book, who lives in the midst of the Chilean Andes, was taught by the "guardians of knowledge" since he was 14 years old. He has been trained among them and belongs to a new generation of Andean Paqos called "citizen bridges," or "Chaca Runes," in the Quechua tongue, the ancient tongue of the "guardians of the wisdom." This book, and the efforts we are making, is playing a leading role in starting to make known the valuable "Andean codes." But also, we will teach the initiations, rituals, and traditions of the millennial wisdom of the Andes that activate the inner centers in each person and bring them into consciousness, and grant knowledge for the modern world of the West.

CHAPTER FOUR

Origin of the "Guardians of Wisdom"

The official history, as taught in history books in Peru, Columbia, Ecuador, Argentina and Chile, is this:

> "The ancestors of the Incas were hunters who came from Asia, crossing the Bering Strait...Groups of those people settled along the way, creating communities." "Others continued south, and between 13,000 BC and 10,000 BC, they reached the Pacific coast of South America and the Andes Mountains, where they settled and found a new way of life."

Some say that the theory is impossible, since no human beings could have traveled so far to get to the Andean mountains, and even more difficult to travel among those endless, iced territories. So, if the theory of the Bering Strait is practically impossible, where do the Incas come from?

Another theory is that the Incas came from Lemuria, the ancient land of "Mu"(Moo), as reported by the archeologist, "Le Plongeon," and by the founder of the "Theosophical

Society," M. Blavatsky. They believed that there was an island in the center of the Pacific Ocean (picture below) that sank into the Ocean after a huge earthquake, more than 10,000 years ago. Le Plongeon and Blavatsky both said that the Lemurians spread their colonies toward Asia, North America and South America. Some of these colonies of Lemuria even traveled so far to the West as to give birth to the first Atlantean colonies.

This theory has not been proven, but contrary to the Bering Strait theory, Lemuria was very close to the Andean mountains. As the map shows below, the distance was much closer than the Bering Strait Theory. But as the "official history" doesn't recognize Lemuria, nor Atlantis, as something factual, they are still strongly attached to the improbable history of the Bering Strait.

Using this Lemurian theory, the pre-Incas of the ancient past, or "the keepers of the wisdom of the ages," after the great earthquake that destroyed their island, sent colonies everywhere, including Asia to the West, (like the Atlanteans mentioned by Plato,) to South America and to North America. These people, who established communities in the Andes Mountains, were known in that place as the

"Children of the Sun," the ancestors of the Incas.

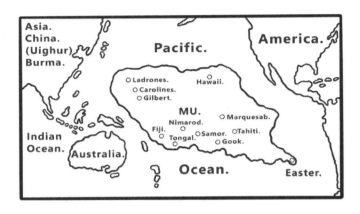

In North America, some Native American Indian tribes, including the Chickasaw and Choctaw, have 'great migration' legends and, as with the Q'eros' reply to Oscar Nuñez del Prado, they were 'Children of the Sun;' the mythologies of the Amerindians' forefathers affirm that they also were Sun Worshippers who, after their land became submerged, travelled across North America from the land of the setting Sun. Additionally, it has been revealed with today's most current information that a Native American man, from the Blackfeet Indian Tribe of Montana, has the oldest DNA native to the Americas. With 99% accuracy, the test revealed the origin of his ancestors' genetics traced back 17,000 years to the Pacific Islands and from there up the South American coast and on to North America. Now is a momentous time to be witness as ancient history reveals a common lineage. With the evident shared ancestry of North and South America, it is appropriate to celebrate the emergence of the Incan prophesy of the Condor, flying with the Eagle; the reunification of South America and North America. This convergence is setting the stage for the return of the Golden Man.

CHAPTER FIVE

Four Levels of Reality

Four Centers of Perception

We are a complex mixture of light and matter, and live simultaneously in four different

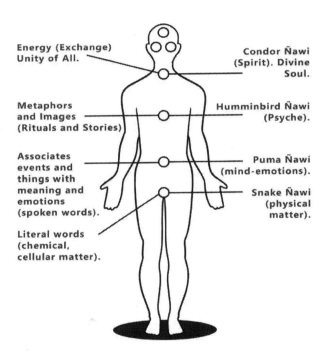

Energy (Exchange) Unity of All.

Condor Ñawi (Spirit). Divine Soul.

Metaphors and Images (Rituals and Stories)

Humminbird Ñawi (Psyche).

Associates events and things with meaning and emotions (spoken words).

Puma Ñawi (mind-emotions).

Snake Ñawi (physical matter).

Literal words (chemical, cellular matter).

Dr. Rod Fuentes
Copyright rodfuentes.org

realities, and each one of them is operating with different laws. For that reason, we do not even know who we are, nor where we're going or what we're looking for in this life.

When we look around us, we see things, people, situations, actions, problems, crimes, violence, and injustices. Since we are a society of rules, we believe that civil laws and religious commandments will help us improve everything around us and solve all our problems. But one of the best examples that this belief and paradigm is completely wrong, is the example of the prohibition of alcohol in the United States during the 1920s.

After being banned by the laws and by churches, people not only continued to drink liquor, perhaps even more than they normally would drink before prohibition. This restriction on people created a powerful network of mafias and organized crime, that struck the United States. There was war between gangsters and gangs, and crimes like never seen before. But this is how we have thought in the past to solve civil and cultural problems, and we continue to believe and think, as a civilization, as a culture in the West, that laws will solve our problems. We have been programmed, or hypnotized, into this belief and life system, even if it fails and doesn't work time and again. It is as if we had, as a society, a bandage placed over our eyes of perception and intelligence; we continue the madness of believing that these unproven methods, which have failed repeatedly, will succeed the next time.

Change the Way You Perceive Reality

The "Guardians of Wisdom" of the Andes, do not live by this bad model for solving their social or personal problems. If they want to change their world, they do not approve new laws or rules. They change the way they perceive their reality; they solve their problems from the highest level of consciousness in a conclusive way. They know and perfectly apply the hierarchy of the different levels of reality to their problems. They know that the lower physical level is governed by the higher mental and emotional level, and that the emotional mental level is governed by the level of the soul, while the highest level of the human soul or psyche is governed by the level of the immortal spirit or Divine Soul. In this way, the "Guardians of Wisdom" solve their problems in one of the levels of reality.

For example, the physical level is usually solved from the mental and emotional level. If it is a problem on the mental and emotional level, they usually resolve it, permanently, from the soul level. And if it is a problem at the level of the soul, they usually resolve it from the Spirit level. From the top level down to the lower levels, they are always solving each situation permanently. And in each of these solutions they always apply them as a basis in everything they did before, during and after the problem arose; because the problems we face must be resolved at the level at which they were created, and it generally corresponds to a higher level than that in which they manifested themselves. If we do it only at the level in which it manifested, and not at the higher level, there will be only a temporary solution, or none at all.

For the "Guardians of Wisdom," the inner centers, called "ñawis," are truly 4 centers of perception, or "observation," that allow them to capture, and be efficient, at each of the 4 hierarchical levels of reality. Each of these centers of perception work in completely different ways from one another, and with different languages. Ñawi means "eye" in the Quechua language, the ancient tongue of the Incas, and the "Guardians of Wisdom" of the Andean mountains.

CHAPTER SIX

Understanding the Four Levels of Reality And Four Centers of Perception

Understanding the 4 levels of reality in which we live, allows us to explain and solve many paradoxes and things in our ordinary life that are very difficult to understand and solve. We will analyze them below. They will allow us to obtain levels of happiness and realization impossible in any other way.

Just as there are four levels of reality, there are four levels of perception through which we come into contact with them. Each of our 4 "perception centers," or ñawis, perceive reality each at its own level, in a unique and particular way, and lives within that reality by sharing the elements of that reality.

The "Guardians of Wisdom" teach that as human beings we live in "four different worlds" of reality and perception simultaneously. When we move from one level of perception to the next higher, we retain our ability to function in the lower levels, but we have a vision or perception quite different from what we are experiencing with the lower levels.

The best example is that of the history of a man encountering three stone carvers. He asks the first: "What are you doing?" and he responds indifferently without even looking at his face: "I'm just carving a stone." The carver was only living and perceiving things from the physical world. When he asks the second, he responds in anger: "Can't you see what I am doing? I do what I have been ordered to do. I have a wife and four children, so I must obey to provide for my family." The second carver is mentally and emotionally interpreting what he does by carving that stone. The causes and purposes of being there, is performing the task. But when he approaches the third stone carver, he verifies that he works with an unusual enthusiasm different from the others. When he asks the same question, the carver responds with joy: "I am building a cathedral." The third carver is perceiving reality from the mystical world of the human soul, the psyche. He works on two levels of perception above the physical, and one level beyond the mental and emotional level. The three are doing the same work in the physical world, but they are perceiving three different realities with their perception, "nawis," (eyes) that work differently.

The same goes for a seller who sells something, for example, cars or watches. The sale will be made from the physical level of the Serpent, showing the physical characteristics of it, simply as a physical product. Or he could do it from the Puma, mental emotional level, associating that car, to status, feelings of freedom, or admiration and power.

This has been understood by the great sales gurus, pointing out that we should not sell "a steak," something physical at the level of the Serpent, but the "smell of the steak," which is something associated with a pleasurable, well-being emotion, that corresponds to the level of the Puma. It is not necessary to show the characteristics or physical features of the product at the level of the Puma, but the benefits or advantages, at the level of the Puma or even the Hummingbird, when acquiring it.

This is clearly represented by the song in the movie <u>Pocahontas,</u> by Disney, showing the differences between the native woman and the English men that arrive with the Virginia Company's expedition to her land. Their goal is to conquer the "new world" with a materialistic thought, at the level of the Serpent, while the native woman sees everything from the level of the Hummingbird or Condor. So, who is the real savage?

She tells him in her song:

"You think you own whatever land, you land on. The Earth is just a dead thing you can claim. But I know every rock and tree and creature, *has a life, has a spirit, has a name."*

(She is perceiving everything from the Hummingbird level.)

"The rainstorms and the rivers are my brothers. *The heron and the otter are my friends. We are all connected to each other, in a circle,* in a hoop that never ends."

(She is perceiving at the level of the Condor that sees everything as interconnected energy.)

In another example, in order to know the sex of a fetus, an ultrasound is called so as to obtain a sonogram. At this point, we are proceeding only at the level of the Serpent, in the physical and material world, but at the highest level, the mystical level of the human soul, we do something much simpler and cheaper. We simply observe the shape of her belly, whether it is pointed or oval.

The Problems We Face Cannot be Resolved at the Same Level at which they were Created.

Being able to move to a higher level of perception can help us to find the understanding and solutions to our problems, that cannot be found in any other way. Knowing this process can help us resolve permanently these conflicts, and cure diseases, and all kinds of other problems, while before we could only perceive anguish and pain. There is a definite solution, usually at a higher level than the physical one, for every problem you encounter in the physical world. You will find a solution for them in your mind, in your emotions, in your subconscious and in your soul or psyche.

You cannot permanently eliminate your monetary shortfalls by just getting another job, if you do not first solve or overcome, your fears of poverty and your bad personal relationships. These problems cannot be resolved at the level at which they were created. You must generally engage the higher level than that in which the problem manifests. If we do it only at the level that it manifested, there will only be a temporary solution, or none at all.

For example, the cause of bad teeth is not only at the physical level caused by too many sugary foods or poor oral hygiene but may be due to the fear of the dentist, or fear of being censored by the dentist. If we do not understand this, we can spend our whole lives taking courses with the greatest and wealthiest of gurus and never resolve our problems, if we do not do it at the level that the problem was created; generally, at the level superior to the physical, at the level of the mind, or of the emotional center, or that of the soul, psyche or the immortal spirit.

We can also spend our entire lives as doctors trying to solve physical illnesses such as cancer, or degenerative or autoimmune diseases. Being mere repairers of bodies, we must solve them at the higher level of the mind, or emotional centers, or from the soul and the Spirit, where these diseases were originally created. Even as a psychiatrist, if we do not understand and seek a true solution at higher levels, trying to solve their mental and emotional problems, we could transform people into drug addicts; that is, the solution will be found on the levels of the soul, psyche or spirit.

CHAPTER SEVEN

More on the Four Centers of Perception in Each Level of Reality

The "Guardians of Wisdom" associate each level of perception with an energetic center, similar to what they call chakra in India, but in the Andes, they are called "Ñawi" in the Quechua language. Ñawi means "eye," and is symbolized metaphorically by an animal that not only represents the restrictions, but also the powers and abilities that one must acquire to grasp and then influence reality from that dimension. Each level also has a language of its own that we must learn to master. Let's look in more detail at each of these levels.

The physical body and the perceptions of the physical or material world are energetically related to the Serpent ñawi. It is an energy center located in the lower zone of the back at the coccyx of our spine and is associated with the black color. It perceives only the realities of the physical world and the body, the organic, the material, the physical events and actions of the first stone carver. Everything is measured at this level of reality in time and space. The physical body is also composed of a part not visible to the eye that is called the etheric body (composed of electromagnetism) or electro vital body. It activates the spinal cord and the primitive reptilian brain. It is the one that evolved from lizards and dinosaurs, and it is a very old and primitive structure that exist fully with force in our central nervous system. In this level of perception and reality, one lives in the physical reality. Its language is literal, material, corporal, chemical, cellular, free of emotions, and sensitivities. It is cold natured and, in many situations, very cruel. It is free from all kindness and sympathy, and completely devoid of emotional intelligence. It is purely an instinctive force.

The Puma ñawi is located at the navel, in the belly, and is associated with the red color. It is linked to the mind, the subconscious and the limbic or mammalian brain. It understands and focuses its attention on the physical world as well. But it interprets the physical world with emotions and sensations, unlike those physical experiences at the level of the Serpent.   The Puma ñawi expresses fear, joy, sadness and a thousand more emotions, and interprets the physical world by giving it a mental and emotional response. To understand what happens in the physical world of man, he uses spoken and written languages, but of an "associative"   type.   Through   these expressions, he makes associations of what happens in the physical world with "feelings," "personal interpretations" and emotions and sensations. At this level, the ego is originated, and subjective interpretations of the outside world are created. We learn what makes us feel good or bad. This level corresponds to the second stone carver, irritable for having to do such heavy work due to his personal circumstances. At this level, what is happening in the physical world in terms of time and space is still measured, but he makes interpretations and adds sensations to what happens in it.

In these two levels of perception and activity, the majority of humanity unfolds and lives. It is in these two lower levels there is a lack of AYNI or Sacred Reciprocity. It is the cold and cruel world of matter, and it is the concrete mind and emotions of a self-centered ego.

In the higher levels appear the birds that fly, the air that allows them to fly is the Ayni or sacred reciprocity, the energy exchange, the giving to others, to all beings, generosity, kindness, compassion and love. In the upper levels the Ayni becomes evident, as it allows these birds the ability to fly towards the higher spiritual regions. Only in those higher levels do the 7 Andean codes begin to operate properly.

In the lower levels of consciousness, the Andean codes may seem fantasies, follies or illusions, and too impractical to be understood and applied by the low levels of the Puma and the Serpent. These animals only move at ground level.

The Hummingbird ñawi, located in the chest, is directly linked to the human soul. It has a much higher mental activity than the Puma and is the true psyche or the human soul. It is associated with a golden color. Its actions activate the neocortex. This level understands the language of the soul, which expresses itself with metaphors, and has a relational language, and archetypal mental visual images. It corresponds to the level of perception of the carver who says, "I am building a cathedral."

At this level of perception, the concept of time and space begins to fade, even though it still exists, but slightly. The concept of "circular time," used by the ancient "Guardians of Wisdom," begins to appear; a concept that has been recently incorporated by the French physicist Jean-Pierre Garnier-Maliet, which he has called "temporary openings" or "unfolding of space and time."

The ñawi, at the perception of the Condor, is located in the throat, directly linked to the Immortal Spirit, associated with a silver color. Its action puts the prefrontal cortex into physical activity. At this level, it works only in the language of the Spirit, which is energy and vibration. In this last level, there simply is no concept of time and space. This level is timeless and non-spatial. It is the world of "unconditioned being" and timelessness.

Here, everything is Ayni, and from this world of the spirit or Divine Soul, the Seven Andean Codes, that will be detailed throughout this book, will be revealed. It is the world of universality, of the unity of all, of pure altruism, kindness, and the noblest of feelings, faith, pure will and legitimate love. It is the highest level of the Divine Soul. It is the Atman or pure soul of the Hindu.

CHAPTER EIGHT

Perception from The Material and Objective Center

The Level of The Serpent

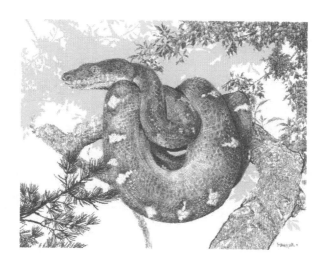

We rely on our physical senses to give us an idea of the material world that surrounds us. Our basic response to the physical world is like the Serpent, because it is completely instinctive. The Serpent has very sharp senses that let her know where there is food. It also easily perceives danger in her surroundings which gives her the ability to survive a predator or hazard in her environment. This is a very material level of perception, where everything is tangible, solid, and where everything is 100% matter, without spirit. Therefore, the conditions of time, space and distance, govern completely at this level, its ability to survive.

So as to quickly flee the place, or fight, the Serpent has a mechanism within its genes to instinctively comprehend situations of physical danger. It is this animal instinct that many people have, at this level of perception, that allows them to avoid physical risk before it occurs, but it should never be confused
with intuition, which corresponds to a much higher level, at the level of the Hummingbird; they are two completely different things that people often confuse.

Likewise, the Serpent has a mechanism of constant self-regeneration and is constantly changing its exterior skin. It represents what is happening in the physical world as it is constantly changing and renewing itself. When observing things from the ñawi, or center of the Serpent, located in the lower part of the spine and associated with the color black, we learn to experience things in such a way that they are not observed in a subjective way, by giving it some personal meaning. At this level of perception of the Serpent's center, events simply happen. Instinct simply acts, there are no feelings of any kind associated with them, neither an analysis, or interpretation, or mental explanation of them. It is simply acting. At this level, the physical events are measurable in time and space; they simply happen at a certain time and in a certain place, without any analysis about it. As the first stone carver objectively answered, "I just carve a stone." He merely describes an action that takes place in a spot, at a certain moment, and nothing more, without interpretations of any kind.

Likewise, it does not rain at the time, in the place where we are staying, to just get us wet, which would be an interpretation at the level of the Puma. It just rains at that time and place. A person does not look at us to make us feel bad, he/she just looks. It's just a physical act, without interpretations, and without sensations or any associated emotions. When this center detects danger, it presents the given situation to the organism and the Serpent is warned immediately.

By learning the perception of this "ñawi," it alters the way in which these experiences have affected us in a subjective and painful way. This is what corresponds to the perceptions at the Puma level and is what we will analyze next. But here we do not give any mental interpretations or emotional associations to things. And more importantly, by experiencing this level of pure perception without contamination, this allows us to free ourselves from the limiting emotional stories we have inherited, or ended up accepting, throughout our lives. We are no longer the cause or effect of anything that happens in the external world, and as we begin to live above this perception, physical things and events just simply happen as a physical phenomenon.

There is a feeling of relief to consciously experience this level of reality, especially if we have lived according to the interpretations to everything on the level of the Puma. In India, certain Exercises[2] have been developed to see and hear without experiencing anything, no thought or sensation, called "tratakum," that teaches us to experience this level of the Serpent and educate ourselves in it.

In the West, we have become accustomed to associate what we see with our own thoughts, and this is one of the most limiting constraints we have; this is equivalent to the ñawi or perception of the Puma in the navel area. When perceiving things from the center of the Serpent, reality is independent of the

---

[2] This book contains extensive exercises to develop the higher levels of reality from where change can be obtained but nothing in this book should be construed for medical advice and the suggestions should NOT take the place of your medical doctor's guidance.

mind and emotions; here there is no emotional intelligence and it doesn't matter what others feel. It is free from the interpretations we make of the things, events and emotions that those interpretations generate within us. It is governed by the instinct of survival. It corresponds to the reptilian brain developed long ago when saber-toothed tigers existed, and people could be devoured by them. It is the physiological or chemical response and how the feeling to flee or fight developed. A large amount of adrenaline is discharged into the blood for this cause, and it generates physical stress for survival.

Along with the survival instinct, another stronger instinct was discovered not long ago by the psychologist Virginia Satir, who said, "Most people think the will to survive is the strongest instinct in human beings, but it isn't. The strongest instinct is to keep things familiar." She considered it even more important than the survival instinct, since many people to whom the external environment, such as the physical or family environment, and the "security" in which they live, when completely changed, end up taking their own lives.

The "Guardians of Wisdom" were initiated in the mastery of the Amaru Serpent. This gave them the skills to activate or deactivate chemicals in their physical bodies and to get complete control of them.

When I was a teenager, I often had dreams of different Serpents, vipers of all kinds, rattle Snake (serpents), and underground caves. This was before meeting Don Joaquin, who opened my eyes to the 4 realities and taught me to look with the 4 perception centers. When I had these dreams, I woke up terrified because the Serpents were very poisonous, huge, thick and disgusting. They were very real in those dreams. They never bit me but the fear of being poisoned by them was frightening.

Now I understand that all adolescents go through a stage where this level of the Serpent becomes manifest to them. This center, or "ñawi," begins to activate at the base of the spine and in the genital area. Especially in the stage of sexual awakening. And at the same time, young boys begin to take on more responsibilities for their material life, something distant for a baby or a small child before adolescence to assume.

The only time this manifestation of the Serpent center before adolescence occurred to me, was when I was about 8 years old. At school they had given us a test that we had to answer in less than 15 minutes. As I delayed answering the questions, the teacher told us that there were only 3 minutes left to deliver the test. I felt a huge pain, which was very intense, in the genital area. It was so painful that I could not bear it and this was the first time I became aware of this survival mechanism in this center.

When I was 14 years old, one of my classmates drowned by falling into the water by a dam that was in the mountains near the area where Don Joaquin lived. Our director, who was a Spanish psychologist, told us that when his body was found, hundreds of meters from where he fell inside the tunnels of the dam, what surprised them most after finding his body, was that he had both hands holding tightly his genitalia. Because of his report, he received a lot of criticism from the public, but he had no explanation.

Don Joaquin explained what had happened to my classmate very clearly. He said, it was because the boy realized that he was within minutes of losing his life, and the survival instinct of the Serpent, located exactly in that area of the body, was set in motion. The classmate's level of understanding is characterized by the absolute impossibility of comprehending the Ayni between the inner being and physical things. It cannot be understood from this level of perception of reality by those who are mentally stuck in the material world, even though the Ayni (Sacred Reciprocity) governs all levels without exception. This level is associated with the underworld or "UJU PACHA" of the Andean wisdom.

Exercises at the Level of the Serpent

Exercise 1.

Look outside your window at a tree, a bush or a person, etc. Look at the tree or person passing by and imagine that this person or object becomes a butterfly. A more dramatic thought makes a better impression. So, imagine that the tree begins to dance. Your thoughts will NOT change what is real, or what is really happening outside.

At the Puma level, we constantly give illusory interpretations to the physical facts, and we begin to live from the mind and emotions, not from the physical reality. If we continue to think about imaginary things that have nothing to do with us, we will begin to think, when looking at ourselves in a mirror, "I am not good enough, I am a bad person, I am unacceptable and an incapable person." We might continue to say these things to ourselves all day, and all our life, which can make that mental illusion a reality. We can also do this with other people or with things.

This day you will begin to separate what you see and hear from the physical reality and from your thoughts; this is called in the East, TRATAKUM. It will make you experience the level of the Serpent, which will be useful for you to counter all negative thoughts about yourself.

Begin by constantly checking your thoughts. Watch them. Do not let them occur by themselves. Do not assume that your thoughts are correct. That's the level of the Puma, with its mental illusions, interpretations and associations, that is expressing itself to you. Until you train the Puma mind, how can you know absolutely that your thoughts are correct? Very often, those thoughts are not even yours; they were introduced into your mind from the outside by other people, teachers, friends, or relatives.

Exercise 2.

Think of something unpleasant about yourself now, that someone has said to you, or that you say to yourself: that you are very fat, that you are very thin, that you are not clever or smart, that you cannot achieve certain things, or that you are not so good, etc.

Hold that thought and mentally take a step back, or to the side, as if you could physically detach from that thought; look at it from the side, or from behind. Look at it from the outside, as if it were an object. Examine it and understand that it is just a thought, just an idea, an idea among millions. It is just as illusory as looking outside your window and imagining that the person walking on the street becomes a butterfly, or that the tree starts to dance. Because you thought it, does not mean it's real.

When you find yourself criticizing yourself, or others, judgments of values, likes and dislikes, pause, an do this same Exercise. When you see objects, only see them as objects, or people as people. Just by paying attention to the physical, and eliminating any thought or feelings attached to them, you will start training the Puma.

This training must be done with consistency. Tratakum was adopted and used therapeutically in the West by Dr. Richard Bandler, with whom I trained, many years ago, as a specialist and Trainer of NLP. It is about analyzing a situation that produces fear or discomfort as if one were seeing oneself on a television screen or imaginary film and in black and white.

This is called "dissociation." In doing so, the person separates the mental interpretations and the limiting emotions of a situation and thus manages to contemplate the objective facts, without emotions whatsoever. This process can change your thoughts and produce a way for a cure for many phobias.

It is about taking something from the subjective and emotional level of the Puma, to that of the emotionless objective level of the Serpent and learn to face those situations from this level of reality. This is what the creators of this discipline, Bander and Grinder, were using to produce different mechanisms of mental dissociations to improve relationships between people who had bad relations with each other; or to accept the criticism of other people, without being affected emotionally by them. All this consists of mentally descending from the mental and emotional level of the Puma, to the objective and physical level of the Serpent. Even though the creators of NLP ignored what they were really doing with these mental Exercises, they have also used the term "different perceptual positions," to name these types of Exercises.

If there is a bad relationship with another person, you can imagine that he is in front of you, a few feet away; then you imagine that you leave your body. Just leave behind your thoughts and emotions and enter the body of the other person. Then you will acquire all his thoughts and emotions, in order to get to understand his world and reality. So, out of your own emotions and thoughts, you begin to see the world from the emotions and thoughts of the other person and begin to understand them better. This is one of the many ways to improve relationships with others; it is quite advisable if this is your practice.

Practice observing yourself on an imaginary screen, like a movie or television movie, a few feet away from you, and watch it in black and white. When you repeat this Exercise many times, you will have learned to separate your mind from the physical situations of emotional attachments. You are moving down from the level of the Puma to that of the Serpent, which in these emotional situations can be very useful.

CHAPTER NINE

The Level of The Puma

Perception from the Mental Center and Subjective Level with Balancing Exercises and Examples

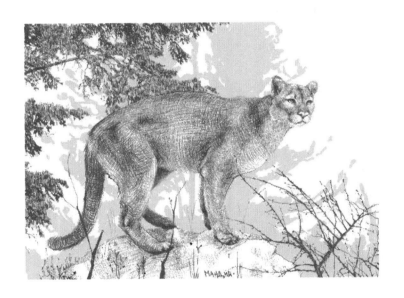

In this level of perception, which is only one higher than the Serpent, we remain very attached to the physical world of matter. But the difference now is that the mind makes thoughts of things, interprets and gives explanations to physical reality, to people, to behaviors, and to physical events. The mind fills them with meanings and emotions.

At this level of perception of the Puma, there is the concrete mind, the lower and material mind, and all its states of emotions, passions, associated with those mental states or thoughts. The lower mind "associates" external things with internal states. It uses an "associative" language that can conclude that two plus two is five. This is something that was detected by the great psychiatrist of the city of Phoenix, Arizona, Dr. Milton Erickson.

For example, at the level of the Serpent, if the survival instinct is activated with physical genital pain, there will be no thoughts associated with that pain, because It is pure instinct. But to experience it from the level of the Puma, that experience is filled with emotions and mental interpretations. At the level of the Serpent, it is identified as a painful sensation in the sexual zone, with possibly a feeling of coldness in the spine. This is what is called the "bristling of the hairs, hairs standing up on the back of the neck, goosebumps, or chills in the spine." If there are very intense sensations, other than fear, such as anxiety, anguish and the like, it can be perceived close to that ñawi, or perception of the Puma, in the mouth, the stomach or solar plexus. There may be nausea or vomiting that is generated at the Puma's mental and emotional level. That which was at the level of the Serpent, only existed as a material phenomenon, without analysis, sensations or emotions. Now, at the level of the Puma, it has a subjective meaning, an interpretation and a feeling associated with it, along with a powerful emotion.

Emotions can be beneficial, such as joy, safety and motivation, or negative, such as anger, anguish, sadness, frustration, doubts and fears. At this level of the Puma, the mechanism of pleasure and pain is also established. We all approach pleasure and flee from pain because of this level.

The concrete mind associates certain external events to these emotions which will then trigger automatically. And, it is good that the concrete mind does this, because it automates a process that should not have to be learned each time, which would be very inefficient. The problem arises when the emotions implanted as automatic responses in the subconscious mind are so limiting that they prevent a normal life and achievements in the higher levels of the Hummingbird and the Condor. At that moment they need to be solved from the same level in which they were created, as I will show later.

Stephen Covey, in his book "The 7 Habits of Highly Effective People," offers an example of how mental meanings determine how we feel or how we act automatically or instantaneously, as fast as the Puma. In his book he tells the story of how some children get on a bus with their father and show a frightful behavior. They move from here to there, they run around, they scream, they play boisterously. People complain to the father about his children's behavior. When he explains that they have just come from the hospital where their mother has just passed away, the people on the bus immediately stop complaining, completely changing their opinion and their emotions and behavior regarding them. We call this, "resignification" and it generates the most rapid, and powerful changes in the mental and emotional states with people and with amazing speed. On this level of perception there arises the saying, "It is not the experience that is important but rather the meaning we give to the experience,"

To have perceptions at this level and to apply quick resignification solutions, as the example in Covey's book, is fully associated with the Puma level, because this type of perception and change can immediately transform situations, making us see them differently right away. The Puma is exactly the correct symbol, and the very archetype of sudden change. The only difference between the level of the Puma, and the level of the Serpent, is that we now make mental and emotional interpretations of things on the physical level. To establish efficiency, these emotional responses become automatic responses in our subconscious mind and get encoded in our personal "luminous energy sphere," or aura. Here, beliefs and emotional conditionings are created that are associated to different events, time and space, and thus the EGO is born. The ego is completely attached to the physical world of external material things, places, events and people. It is responsible when happiness is taken from us. The ego is offended if someone speaks ill of us, or if someone says things that we do not agree with, which can lead to anger and hatred.

In the tradition of the "wisdom of the Andes," that which is related to a "personal energy sphere," or "energy bubble," is a manifestation of the four levels of reality, mixed one to another, as we will see later. This sphere completely surrounds our body and, in the West, it has been called the aura. The Andean "Guardians of Wisdom" call it "luminous energy sphere," or POQPO.

When we have limiting or negative emotions like anger, frustration, sadness, and hatred, *the energy of this personal sphere experiences stagnation.* A kind of mud or stagnant energy appears in certain areas of the aura, and over time it can give rise to various diseases. So, from the level of emotion, this stagnant energy descends, or manifests, later on at the physical level of the Serpent, as a disease. These diseases also dissolve physically, in a definitive way, only when the mental and emotional interpretations that we associate with them are also dissolved. In the following paragraphs you will see how to do it using an example of the physical effects it had on a woman.

For the "Guardians of Wisdom," the ego normally manifests itself under three falsities: illusions, deceptions or masks. The ego may also take on the persona of three figures: the victim, the executioner or the savior. Through the mask of the victim, the ego seeks satisfaction by becoming irresponsible of itself, not caring what happens to it, living fully on a platform of "necessity" and weakness; while accusing or blaming others for everything bad that happens to her.

Then the role of the executioner appears, always angry with everyone because everyone is to blame for their problems. It is a violent extension of the victim. Again, she is not responsible for herself, nor does she care what happens to her. She lives fully in a platform of "need" and weakness, blaming others for her miseries.

And finally, the most illusory of all roles is that of the "savior," where the ego is considered so important that it comes to take responsibility for others, through her help, they become dependent on her, with the excuse that they need her to reach salvation. The "savior" points out, that without her help, they do not have the possibility of saving themselves. It is enthroned in this way, with a very deceptive disguise, making them dependent. To make others fall into their physical and emotional dependence, the "savior" can use the figure of a "healer," a psychic, a channeler, a leader, or politician, a teacher, a master initiate, or a guru.

The Puma's instincts are different from those of the Serpent, the latter only worries about sexual reproduction, survival and physical security. Cougars are curious and inquisitive, and because of this, our feline instincts lead us to the right or wrong people, beliefs and situations; the latter, if this instinct is deficient. The perception of the Puma is associated with the mammalian or limbic brain, the brain of emotion and equally with that of intimacy, empathy and pleasure; or hate, antipathy, aversion and disgust. It can also generate superstition.

When you see a beautiful woman or handsome man, you will notice their smile, the symmetry of their face, their eyes and hair and their figure. These purely physical observations are at the level of the Serpent, which would induce an attraction, or desire, that you find very pleasurable. Such feelings produce a mental image, or a hallucination, of dominating or surrendering to this person of the opposite sex. You are dazzled by the desire to be with this person, until awakening to the misery and suffering of being at the mercy of another human being was due to our lust. However, at the level of the Puma, it would produce the idea of beauty and perfection, which would create a feeling of love and an emotional attraction beyond the physical desire of lust. But, when we are charmed at the level of the Puma, we are able to use subjective associations and become dazzled by beautiful words, false promises and persuasions of swindlers. Because we have more possibilities at this level than at the Serpent, we are able to make effective changes and solve much more complex problems that will enrich our life.

By building great myths and illusions about reality, the ego, with all its attention turned to the outside, establishes the belief that happiness is in external things. The term ego can be deceptive, because when we say ego, it sounds as if we are talking about a person, a child or something real. Essentially, the ego is a "little idea" about our individual being, and the idea is: everything good is outside. The ego is always very conditioned and convinced that everything depends on the exterior, on things, places, objects or people. This is subjecting something as intangible as happiness to the physical world and one can become deceived with this terrible fantasy. The ego is responsible for individuality, for competitiveness, and for the separation of people in different groups that fight and struggle. It is exactly contrary to what is lived at the level of the Condor, which is: unity, cooperation, help, Ayni and the golden rule.

At this ego level, the activities and contents of the courses and seminars of personal development, self-help and coaching, even the same Exercises taught in this book about the level of the Hummingbird, can be dwarfed, distorted and corrupted, and so transform those good ideas into evil. Since the ego cannot understand the principle of AYNI, it will not support those contents and teachings. Personal development, acquired power, well-being and even physical health, can become evils for other people, when the ego rules, because it completely lacks a healthy understanding of sacred reciprocity. To make the ego bigger, it uses prosperity to take advantage of others, and personal power to impose itself on the weakest. Because of the power of the ego, someone can make amazing sacrifices to become a powerful healer, or magi, and once accomplished, they can do more harm than good to their fellow man. All this happens at the level of the Puma.

The level of the Puma makes a completely subjective interpretation of its reality, and when it is very deficient, it can also lead to very limited mental and emotional pathologies. We can create on this level, with our beliefs and subconscious conditioning, a true network of mental illusions, or a true "mental matrix" that completely envelops our existence. But also, the mind can give correct interpretations, and realize that a disease can be created by the mind, and that the positive mind and emotions can equally restore health.

At this level, unlike the Serpent, you can repress anger or resentment which can cause serious illness, while a positive attitude can bring joy and peace to ourselves and those around us. The physical world and what happens here has an explanation and a meaning created by us or borrowed from others in whom we place our trust. We are aware that our experiences are influenced by our thoughts, and that everything is not necessarily as it seems to be in the literal or visible physical world. At this level, there is a strong attachment to time and space.

Childhood, adolescence, youth, maturity and old age are not only physical, cellular, and a physiological phenomenon; we grant them a mental and emotional meaning, subjectively determined by us at this level. Only the concepts of the concrete mind are understood at this level. It is not possible at this level to understand the operation of intuition or abstract laws that corresponds to the upper level of the Hummingbird. The Puma level is the plane of emotional associations, envy and jealousy. The theft of intelligence and information are very common among those who use this level, especially with academics. The pain we experience at the level of the Puma is no longer just physical or chemical; here, we add something incomprehensible, as we begin to know emotional pain and mental suffering. As demonstrated by Dr. Dave Dobson, a famous American hypnotherapist, this type of suffering can be greater than the physical pain and can even make the physical pain increase, or decrease, and even disappear, using only thoughts and words. This is possible because an immediately superior level of reality influences and governs on this lower level. On the upper level you can solve or create the problems that will manifest in the lower level.

After having passed through adolescence with all those dreams about Serpents and vipers, I began to become aware of the center of the Puma, when my dreams changed to wild animals, such as bears, wolves, jaguars, tigers, lions and pumas. But also, vampires, a kind of "undead" with fangs, like tigers, lions, wolves and bears. I remember a very powerful and frightful dream where a lion ran through the interior of a house, devouring those who were inside. And, another, of a tiger devouring people; I heard the bones of the victims being crushed by the jaws of the tiger, inside a closed park. It was truly a metaphor for my subconscious mind, a terror of being dominated at this level, that can make our life a "locked house," because a feline doesn't share with us the true life that is behind its doors. These dreams are warnings, regarding the need to understand these levels of our reality. Dreams, of vampires attacking with their fangs, add the ideas of the "living dead," the cemetery and stagnation. They all correspond to the idea of being stuck on this level, in a superficial or frivolous and vain life, filled with erroneous mental interpretations of existence, and disturbed emotions, a true living death as a result of them. Similar to the other levels, except for the Condor, this level has a bright and a dark side. On its dark side it can make our life hell.

In the immortal work of John Bunyan, **The Pilgrim's Progress**, there´s a metaphor of the Pilgrim, who advances towards the City of the Light, where God is. But on his way, he must cross a path where he will meet wild beasts, that seek to devour him. The most atrocious thing that can happen to people who live *only* at the level of the Serpent and the Puma, is disintegration of the physical body at death; but not so for those who live at the level of the Hummingbird and Cougar. Buddhists try to free people from this pain, by having them build beautiful mandalas, and then destroy them. But there is a less violent and better way than that: by simply developing the levels of perception and awareness at the level of the Hummingbird and Condor. At the level of Cougar and Serpent, one can understand only intellectually the AYNI between beings and things. This spiritual concept can only be understood by the concrete mind, but it will be a principle to which the ego will try to profit or benefit selfishly. The ego will only have selfish interest in the forces of AYNI, or simply will not believe in it and will live completely immersed in the ego and selfishness, which is exactly the opposite.

The AYNI governs at all levels, which does include the Puma. If we are kind, kindness will be given to us; if we are cold and selfish, we will receive the same in return. This level is associated with the natural world or KAI PACHA of the Andean people.

Exercises at the Level of the Puma

Exercise 1. Working with a Partner

If you can work with a partner or friend, ask him/her to stand in front of you, and then give you three different severe criticisms. "You are very…."

These must be powerful criticisms. Listen to those words but stay completely indifferent to them. When listening to these words or "grievances," observe and feel how these criticisms try to awaken emotions. These feelings are the conditionings of the Puma level, from which you must free yourself day by day.

The solution is to divide them into three parts:

First, with the previous Exercises of Tratakum, or dissociation, *descend* to the level of the Serpent.

Second, heal the situation at the Serpent level by obtaining valuable lessons, or by doing a "re-meaning," which I will teach below.

Third, *ascend* to the top level of the Hummingbird and transform everything into metaphors and teachings for the benefit of your spiritual being; this will be analyzed at the Hummingbird level, below.

Exercise 2. Controlling Emotions

The key to the emotional domain is to understand what each emotion was initially designed for, by the concrete mind, at the level of the Puma and learn to understand its initial purpose. Learning emotional control, at the level of the Puma, in general, is a really important step to being successful in life. When there are obstacles in life, this one thing will prevent you from giving up. If things start to go wrong, it's the only thing that will give you an early warning system. But your intellect, your normal mind, which decades ago initially programmed the emotion into your subconscious mind and sphere of luminous energy, *has not yet reached an understanding of what is happening*. Essentially, when interpreting the world as good or bad, the emotions that originated in the concrete mind, for functional efficiency, left that emotion imprinted at the level of the subconscious. Subsequently, in front of the appropriate trigger, emotions will arise from the subconscious, which I call the "sticker" of emotions or states. From deep within us, these emotions will not have the rational mind intervening. It will be a kind of early warning signal to tell you how things are going, according to how that emotion was programmed by your mind in the past. It will tell you if your life is on the right track or not, corresponding to the interpretation that was made of that experience in the past. This is what joy, excitement and other like emotions are all about. It will also point out when things are going wrong, if initially such experience was qualified by your concrete mind as bad or harmful in the past. As mentioned, these experiences are programmed into your subconscious as well; this is the reason for the appearance of stress, fear, anxiety, and doubt.

All these states are emotional responses from your subconscious that ask you to pay attention.

The problem is that if people ignore their emotions or bury them, then they will come back in some way. Either the pressure will grow until it explodes, or it will return to bite you later at the most inopportune and unexpected moment. In terms of your biochemistry, in terms of how you feel inside, there is very little difference between excitement and fear. The big difference is in your mind, it's how your concrete mind interprets those signals, or how you programmed that response in the past. When you think of possible harm, "excitement" becomes fear, and it makes you anticipate even worse things. This is the reason why the same situation can make some people feel totally excited and thrilled, say when riding a roller coaster, and other people are totally terrified. There really is no difference in the experience beyond what the mind is interpreting. The fear we perceive is the result of what we do with it inside our mind or the interpretations and meanings that our mind gives to certain experiences. When our boss shouts at us, or when someone is angry at us, or when someone threatens us, our mind interprets it in a way that will cause us fear, or anger. So, our perceptions and how we see the world, how we understand what is happening, are a crucial ingredient in how we are going to feel. This is how emotions arise.

An event happens, you perceive it, you notice it consciously, or unconsciously, in the inner mind. Now, inside yourself you have certain beliefs and perceptions of how the world works, and a part of you is going to think "oh," when such and such happens, so I will do this or that thing. Your mind is interpreting the meaning of the situation. That moment of meaning, that value judgment, that sense of this or that, and what is happening is crucial. As a result, you realize what that event means, or rather you start to think about what it means, and a good or bad emotion will arise. It is completely encoded in your sphere of luminous energy from the past, as well. If in your concrete mind it means something positive, then you will feel fantastic; but if it means something negative like anger, fear, sadness or doubt, all these dark emotions begin to appear. How do people usually deal with their negative emotions? Many people, who only live at the level of the Serpent, may seek an anxiolytic, or any other physical solution, like drinking alcohol, smoking, or going out to do Exercises, taking a bath in warm water or just relaxing. Some people watch television and eat chocolates or ice cream, which is also a kind of physical medication to mask the emotion, until the moment passes, and we feel good again. That is, they seek to do something physical that distracts their attention from something else, which can lead to all kinds of behaviors. It is not the most efficient movement, because a solution at the level of the Serpent will only be able to superficially calm the emotion, but it will not dissolve and cure it. It will probably produce side effects, and it can generate alcoholism, obesity, addictions or dependence on drugs. Remember, you must go to the level where it was created, which is the mental and emotional level of the Puma.

At this level, people try to do many things, the first and most common is to simply suppress and ignore the emotion. An emotion appears, you do not like it, you push it away, you push it deeper inside and you say "no, I will not have this in my life," and with all your willpower, you turn it off. Sometimes, suppressing an emotion momentarily is the right thing to do. Let's say you're a father and your child does something that arouses anger. You do not necessarily want to jump up and down, yell at him and call him horrible names, because that's not a good thing to do to a child. It's okay to keep that emotion under control for a while until you can investigate what is really happening. You can solve this by an efficient method that I will teach.

The real key at the level of the Puma is to solve all emotions and not to suppress them, but to understand the lessons that they contain. If you learn the lesson, the emotion will naturally be released, and your work will have been done. You will hear the message it contained so that you can move on, and once the lesson is understood, it will not return. But remember, emotions are a sign of early warning, and if you ignore them, you can bet on one thing: *they will come back stronger*. So, the key to controlling your emotions is to discover what that message is, to read the message and to find out what you need; in that moment, the emotion will go away. The emotion will say "very well, then I'll leave, and I'll leave you alone." This is something that you will want to do because the emotions will give you very valuable information about the moment when they were created by your concrete mind and imprinted an energy code in your "energy bubble" or POQPO. The things that we normally do not pay attention to will emerge subconsciously through your emotions and by being able to release them you will learn many things about yourself and the world around you that will help you.

How are we going to begin to interact with our emotions, at the level of the Puma, in a different way, so we don't suppress them, but liberate them, and carry out the lesson that it contains? I will give you 9 simple steps you can follow to get it done. Once you have mastered these nine steps you will have the key to the control of emotions at the level of the Puma.

Exercise 3.   Locate the physical sensation.

Remember, all emotions are a combination of two things, a *physical sensation* inside the body, with meaning, and *judgment* about that sensation that has been felt; it is the meaning that your concrete mind gave to the experience in the past. So, the first step is to discover where does this come from? This is not as easy as it seems. Some people can do it instantly, but others, when you ask them, "Are you angry now, how do you know?" They will tell you "I do not know." Where do you feel anger? "Everywhere." Most likely, they do not feel it everywhere. They could have a tension in their chest. They might feel something in the pit of the stomach. Maybe their hands are tingling. Maybe the temperature is rising in the face or maybe their face feels hot and red.

Some people find it more difficult to work with emotions. In fact, they have become very efficient at eliminating their emotions. In general, it is a way to cope with very strong emotions that they would not know how to handle at that moment. However, now that you know how to handle your emotions, you need to be able to get back in touch with them, because that security mechanism, that blanket of suppression that you set, should go away forever. If you are really going to start releasing all the things that have been accumulating below, you must deal with them. So, if for some reason you have trouble locating the actual physical experience of that emotion, do not worry, there is a simple Exercise that you can do to be more and more in tune with your body and feelings. Try it now.

The first thing to do is scan your entire body for a moment, from head to toe and observe your chest, your hands, your feet, your legs, your knees, your back, the top of your head, your face and so on. Observe every part of your body and the sensations that are there when that emotion is present.

→ You may have an itching sensation.
→ You may have a gurgling in the stomach.
→ It is possible that you have a heat that develops in one hand but not in

the other.

→ You can have a foot that feels restless.

→ You may have a part of your body that feels more relaxed or tense.

What you are looking for now is any sensation. Basically, start telling your subconscious mind, I'm going to start paying attention to these things now, so, you can start revealing to me more and more of these sensations until it becomes a habit. If you're the kind of person who does not find it easy to get in touch with your emotions, then the sensations in your body will be an excellent place to start. Go ahead and do it.

Maybe you'll spend five, ten minutes every day scanning your body and noticing, "Oh, I have a tight stomach now that I did not know was there before. My shoulder blades, yes, they are also sore and maybe I feel something in my stomach, and I cannot say what it is yet." It's okay. So, now you are learning to locate sensations within your body. Then, when you start having difficulties, in real life, for example, when there is an emotional problem or a situation where you feel overwhelmed or scared, you will be more experienced interacting with your own body to locate where the source originates, where it is it radiating or what is the source of these feelings.

Exercise 4.
Begin to interact with that feeling.

Remember that there is a message, put there by your concrete mind in the past, within your subconscious. This message is somewhere, and you are trying to find out where it is. The way to do this is very simple. You will start to find a label or a name that matches the experience. Usually, it will not be the first thing that will occur to you. For example, it may feel like an oppression or a buzzing sensation in the pit of your stomach. You might tell yourself that it's something like fear, but it's not quite scary, or you may not be totally sure about the feeling.

This is exactly what needs to be done.

Why? Because what you're doing is starting to label the feelings, and once you put a word, or a label with the feeling, you're going to check again with the emotion and analyze it. Is that name the right one? Is that the correct label? Maybe you answer: "Yes, but not quite sure." What is missing? "Well, it's a kind of emotion that is mixed with fear. So, I'm kind of excited and scared at the same time. This is a bit weird." But when you say that, "it's fear and another emotion at the same time," there will be a change. If you have a label close enough, the sensation begins to transform. Maybe it moves in the body, or maybe it diminishes in intensity. You are changing an unconscious process into another conscious one. It may change essentially in its very nature, because many emotions are layered one on top of the other.

The key here, and this is very important, is that you should observe the experience, instead of getting involved with it. *Because you are transforming an unconscious process into another conscious one, getting involved with it spoils it.* For example, let's assume it is fear. When people feel afraid, they try to get away from this emotion. It is the whole issue of the "flee or fight" mechanism, only this time we are trying to flee from ourselves, from our own experience, instead of from outside things. The problem with this is that if you start talking about fear, saying, "it's because my grandmother just yelled at me." Or, "it's because I hope this is going to happen," you're starting to create a story about what may or may not be accurate; this begins an error at this stage. All you want to do at this stage is simply *observe* it as a scientist. "Oh, look, the body is experiencing this, this is interesting."

Exercise 5. Do not fight the experience.

Do not try to push it away. You're not trying to do anything with this emotion, yet. You are simply trying to realize what is really happening and see if you can find a label that matches the emotion. There is a general rule that you will want to follow, called "what resists persists." What you accept, you can transform, and this is a true key to everything. The situations that you resist, will tend to persist and will grow and escalate. If you accept them, as they are now, you will have the power to begin to transform them, changing them by going with their nature instead of going against it.

Nine Techniques of Emotional Release at the Level of the Puma

1. Find a sensation inside your body from some situation that generates a negative emotion.

2. Label it, that is, give it a name
Observe how you feel. What is it? Is it fear? Is it another emotion? Is it anger? Is it sadness? What would you call it? Even if you cannot put a label on it, call it "fuzzy or round, or red." This is part of the process, too.

3. Keep watching the changes that occur when doing it.
When you tag it, check with your feelings again and see what happens now. Has it changed? So, what is it now? "Well, the emotion or feeling of fear has now changed into something like anger. It's a bit of anger with a bit of sadness too."

4. Do not fight against it.
Points four and five are closely related.

5. Do not fight just watch it.
Do not fight against the experience, just observe it and allow yourself the freedom to experience that emotion for a moment so that you can begin to break free.

6. Start learning the lessons.

Allow the lessons to come on board.
This will become relatively natural once you begin to find the root of this emotion; in other words, how your concrete mind formed it in the past. If you feel a sensation, you put a label on it, change it a bit, put on another label and change it a little bit and then pay attention to everything else that happens. Suddenly, an image may appear in your mind, for example, when someone shouted at you 10 years ago and you ask yourself, "why did I think about that?" You are finding the moment when your concrete mind made the interpretation of the physical world for the first time related to this experience, at the level of the Puma, and put that meaning and associated emotional response in your subconscious. The reason you thought about that is because that event in the past is related in some way to this current event and emotion, and you can verify it if you want. You can ask yourself, "when that teacher shouted at me 20 years ago, was it related to this?" Something changes, it's like a recognition, and your subconscious mind says, "you're listening, I finally got your attention".

Now you want to learn those lessons. You will learn if this meaning was incorrect at that time. You can change that meaning now that you are older and wiser. You begin to acknowledge what is happening, and finally the whole experience begins to change, and the emotion is released; It was trapped, but now it gives you an account of the meaning associated with it. This is technically called "re-signification." At that time, perhaps the meaning you gave was of high intolerance and the lesson might be that you need to be more tolerant. You cannot have such high expectations of other people. The lesson might be that you need to put more limits on your life, it is not good to let people walk over you, and much more.

7. Apply the lesson or "re-signify". Now that you know when the emotion originated, and now you also know the meaning that your concrete mind gave to certain experiences in the past, which act automatically from your subconscious today as negative emotions. Now you must make a commitment to make sure that what you have learned from this will help you to change it. Otherwise, you will not have learned anything at all, and you will not have improved anything from the level of the Puma.

Let's say you've been frustrated lately. Then you locate that physical sensation contained in the emotion, and it's like somewhere in your stomach and maybe a little lower, and it's a tension with energy inside of it. You still cannot label it at all, but you're watching it, you're leaving it there and suddenly you understand, it's like a tension, like frustration. That's what it is, it's like a frustration. The feeling changes. Something else happens. Maybe now there is a bit of anger, and suddenly an image appears in your mind of your friend and you say, "this is weird, why did I think of my friend?" The sensation now changed into something more like anger. When contemplating that, suddenly you can have the sensation of an idea, an epiphany, or awareness. You are finding the original meaning that your concrete mind put on that event years ago, perhaps as a child. Maybe a voice tells you, it speaks to you inside, or maybe you have this feeling inside, and it gives you the feeling that, "yes, all these things that my friend has been asking me to do, are extreme. I mean, he is really starting to want too much in terms of what he expects me to do for him." Suddenly, you realize that you are being used as a doormat by that person and that is the lesson, but to learn it, you must do something else about it. Some things do not really require real action. Some things only require you to see things differently, and go to a level higher, that is, go to the level of the Hummingbird.

Let's analyze this frustration, and let's say that the frustration is because you have a friend that struggles to get ahead, but it does not work for you, but you really want him to be successful. Maybe the lesson is that you cannot interfere in the lives of other people. Let them make their own mistakes. Let them have the freedom to learn from their own mistakes. At that point, you must develop more tolerance, it is no longer your "dumb friend," rather, it is your lovely friend who is making his way in life.

So, the lesson is not so much to know what is happening, but to perceive the situation in another way, to realize that every time your "foolish friend" makes a mistake, it is not a mistake that he is committing, it is an opportunity for him to learn something. Now, generally, you can help him learn something, instead of trying to force him to do the right thing. Your friend is really on the path of a spiritual evolution.

*If you take this step correctly, you will automatically go to Step 8.

8. Experience a true release.

The emotion will simply evaporate. In general, it is a kind of energy emission because the energy is still inside your "luminous energy sphere." But instead of getting caught and trying to get your attention with its message, it is now released. You will have liberated that energy.

*The final step is very simple. In fact, you have already done it.

9. Scan your body once more to check that it is clear.

If there's still something there, like a scolding in the background, you can say to yourself, "Okay, I guess I have most of it, but there's still something else that I have to deal with." Perfect, if you face it now, fantastic; if you decide you're going to do it later, it does not really matter, because now you are building a relationship with your subconscious that reflects the codes in your "sphere of luminous energy," placed there by your concrete mind, at the level of the Puma (mind and emotions). With time, the more you do this, the more natural it becomes for you, the more things are resolved and often this happens completely automatically.

Now I would like you to realize something. Just because you're doing these Exercises does not mean you're going to have an instant hit every time. Some things need to be worked on with persistence. For example, occasionally you might have an argument with someone, and you go home and start thinking about it. Instead of imagining different scenarios of, "I should have said this," or "I should have said that," etc., you begin to pay attention to the emotions and perform this liberation Exercise. By doing so, you can learn a lot about yourself, and the interaction with your friends, or relatives, so that you become aware of what you are angry about?

The problem is sometimes caused when we are in the heat of an emotion, and we attribute it to something very wrong. Maybe they dropped the fork, picked it up, and kept eating with it. Then you say, "How unpleasant, it is horrible that she is doing this, she is an unpleasant and disgusting person." That's honestly what you might be thinking at the time, but that may not be the real problem. Maybe it is that you have so many expectations of that person that you cannot allow her to make any mistakes, and if she makes mistakes, you get angry with her. Maybe you're ashamed to be with that person in public. *You begin to realize that it has more to do with who you are, than with what the other person is doing.* So, instead of starting the fight again, and telling them why and what, you can better grow and learn from it as a person. In other words, you become more tolerant in a situation, or maybe you talk to that person about the different ways of interacting with you so that the relationship is transformed into one that is good for both of you. Now you will be solving genuine problems instead of just reacting and doing the first thing that comes to mind, which is not always correct. Now you have an alternative to getting stuck at the level of the Puma; now you have a solution.

These are the nine steps of the technique of *emotional release and learning*, from the level of the Puma. Practice with persistence this excellent method that I developed to have mastery of this level; it will bring you abundant and wonderful fruits.

CHAPTER TEN

Experiences at the Puma Level

An example of Healing of a Chronic Disease at the Level of Mind and Emotions

... A woman who suffered from rheumatism, visited a doctor.

After examining the inflamed joints of her hands, he asked:

"How long have you been afflicted?"

"Since I was 17 years old," she replied.

"Who did you get angry with about 18 or 19 years ago?" the doctor asked again.

"With my older brother," the patient said. "I was so angry with him that I left home, and I have never spoken to him since then."

"Then," the doctor said, "go and make peace with your brother, forgive him for everything he has done, and then return to me for treatment."

The patient went to her brother's house and, to her surprise, was welcomed with open arms. She told him that she regretted it and was sorry for everything that had happened between them. Her brother told her that everything was fine and that he never had any resentment against her. She was so happy for her brother and her family that she stayed at her brother's house longer than she had expected.

Back home she thought to stop and visit the doctor to tell him that she no longer needed his services. All the pains, hardness and inflammation of the joints had completely disappeared. The doctor smiled and explained: "I knew you would be fine, when you had completely and wholeheartedly forgiven your brother."

Real examples of not practicing "Sacred Reciprocity" Selfishness instead of AYNI

Example 1

Bob is a person quite close to the author of this book, who had heard about the AYNI, but really did not believe in this principle. He lived only from the level and perception of the Puma, which was from his ego. Because he was the owner of an industry of recognized fame, in the national environment of his country, he sought to publicize its products massively. A friend of his, who was the commercial manager of a television channel, offered to put an advertisement on air at a very low cost. It was a personal favor and an arrangement "between friends." Nobody had control over the commercial manager, and everything would work out very well. Nobody would find out. It was an advantage that the manager made from his position of power and control at the TV station. No contract would be signed, nor would the fees for the services of the television channel be documented. Everything was fine up to there, however, the director of the television channel made a change of personnel and the friend of Bob, the commercial manager, was dismissed.

After the ads had been published, the Channel began to charge Bob the fees he owed, which, even though it was a very low cost, he had not paid from the beginning. He denied everything, demanding to be shown the fees he had to pay and the existence of a contract, which he knew did not exist. The Channel did not accept the explanations given by Bob and executed a series of moral pressures, so that he would pay his commercial obligations. Bob smiled, satisfied, because "legally" nothing could be done against him. Simultaneously, Bob began to have problems with some of his employees in his industry and was sued in court.

Bob was summoned to court and, despite having the best lawyers he could afford, the

Judge imposed an "agreement" between the parties, for an amount of money equivalent, only a little higher, to the amount that he should have legitimately paid for the advertising at the TV Station. Coincidence? NOT from the perspective of the teachings of the "Guardians of Wisdom."

Now that Bob signed the compromise to pay for the "agreement" offered by the Judge, "coincidently," the pressures of the executives of the television Channel ceased immediately. They simply informed the directors of the Channel that it was an "uncollectible account." From that moment, Bob took very seriously the teachings of the "Guardians of Wisdom," especially that related to the "Sacred Reciprocity," or Ayni.

Example 2

I have seen the fall of a successful entrepreneur, who based his success solely on taking advantage of the ignorance of others. He made unfavorable deals, did not fulfill his commitments, and postponed the payment of wages, without justification. By taking advantage of others, he personally gained and made money from his costumer's bank interest. In a few years, all his material "empire," and his happiness, vanished like a puff of smoke. It was the cumulative effect of all his deficits with the Ayni or "Sacred Reciprocity."

I have also seen a lawyer, that rendered negligent and careless services to his clients, which completely ruined the client. His goal was only personal and selfish: just for profit. He didn´t care about anyone else, or the quality of the services. Taking a clue from the downfall of the entrepreneur mentioned previously, can you imagine what happened to this lawyer's business?

To be in good compliance with the Ayni, we must be quite generous in all areas of our life. Be very careful in your obligations, duties and responsibilities. Be extremely careful in assuming some type of contract or compromise on your word. You must comply fully with all agreements and promises. Be extremely careful to compensate duly those who are under your responsibility or provide you with labor or services. If you want something, be it prosperity, love or friendship, and you give generously these things to others, they will return to you multiplied, because of the Ayni. And besides, as a special bonus, you'll enjoy an inner satisfaction, or happiness, that is impossible to achieve in any other way.

CHAPTER ELEVEN

The Level of the Hummingbird

Perceptions from the Upper Mental Center

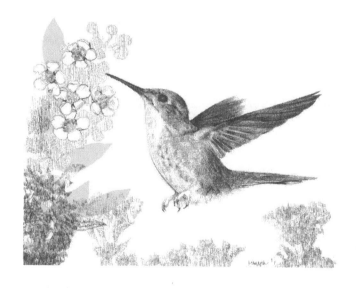

The level of reality and perception of the Hummingbird is that of the higher mind, or that of the Psyche. The ancient Greeks represented the Psyche with the Butterfly. Some also called the Hummingbird level the "human soul," to distinguish it clearly from the next level; the

Condor level, called the "Divine Soul." The Hummingbird is the level of the superior capacities of the mind such as ideals, imagination, faith, optimism, the abstract, the unknown, the mythical and magical. At the level of the Puma, the mind is placed in the world of matter, the tangible, and at the level of the Hummingbird, the mind is placed in the intangible, and what is not seen with the physical eyes. Hence, having wings, the Hummingbird no longer crawls on the ground like the Serpent and the Puma. There is an aspiration towards what belongs to the world of the Condor, the magical, and the spiritual. Unlike the two lower levels, here we find the first animal that flies, or rises, in the air. Just as a person can have dreams about Serpents, or wild beasts, which represent the first two levels of perception of reality, when someone has dreams where he flies, it is a signal, or call, to begin to develop perception at these higher levels of reality.

I remember having told my relatives about my childhood dreams where I flew through the skies, over buildings, rivers and valleys; they laughed at me for being so "imaginative. " It is the same thing those, who live only at the level of the Serpent and the Puma, say about people who start living in the reality of the Hummingbird. The language of this level of reality and perception is constituted mainly by music, poetry, meditations, images, and dreams. It is the realm of myths, where the human soul, known as "manas" in the Hindu tradition, can experience itself on a magical, divine or sacred journey. It is here where the mind no longer governs the essential, concrete, or logical thoughts and moves from the world of the Puma. At the level of the Hummingbird we find the superior thoughts of faith, including intuition, the abstract, the will, creativity, hope, and the magical which fosters feelings that assume an important role in our lives. The Hummingbird is the level of the intuitive geniuses, of Einstein, Tesla, Leonardo Da Vinci, Galileo and Mozart; and of sciences, the arts and mythology.

At the level of the Hummingbird, unlike what we cannot solve with the concrete and analytical mind of the Puma, we can solve problems quickly, with just one glimpse of inspiration. It is equivalent to what has been associated with the activity of the right hemisphere of the brain, which is noted for reading body language, the abstract, symbols, archetypes and the art of dance. Although it is very small, this little bird is capable of flying thousands of miles alone, without a flock like other birds. The Hummingbird is full of confidence, faith and hope in its journey, even in the face of the unknown. Most notable is the fact that Hummingbirds' habits have been tracked and they are able to find their way back to the same house, to the backyard of that same house, without cartography or modern technology; this is a feat that many experienced commercial airline pilots would consider extremely difficult to carry out. How do they do that? The *Source of Everything*, the necessary knowledge, has been put inside the little Hummingbird, so it can perform these feats. To inspire us as human beings, Mother Nature has created and formed this tiny bird in a remarkable way. In the realm of the mythical, we are all like true Hummingbirds, on a great journey, with a desire to drink of the divine, just as the Hummingbird drinks the nectar of life from flowers that the Mother has provided.

When we perceive our life as something magical or divine, it means that we are living at the level of the sacred Hummingbird. Here, at this higher level, we begin to detach ourselves from the ideas of time and space and physical measurements, and circular time begins to appear on the horizon of our minds. Things begin to become less defined in terms of measurements. We begin to enter the world of universal archetypes. Time, distance and the concept of separation begin to disappear; it begins to vanish altogether on the upper level of the Condor. Otherwise, we are stuck in the level of the Puma, that of the concrete mind and its lower mind interpretations of the physical world.

From the Hummingbird level, we see all our experiences as part of a magical, divine and extraordinary journey, as something sacred, and divine. The perceptive state of the Hummingbird is associated with the neocortex and to it we owe the ability of intuition. It is also the language of the metaphor of healing images, of healing visualizations, and of visual metaphors, that awakens the mind to realities not understood by the concrete mind at the lower level. These stories and metaphors serve as the relational languages of nature, giving sustenance to the human soul.

At this level, the French neurophysiologist and Hermetic, Dr. Gerard Encausse, understood the complete structure and nature of a human being by observing a carriage being pulled by a horse. Watching an apple fall from a tree, Newton understood the existence of a law of universal gravitation. Equally, at the level of the higher mind or human soul, or Hummingbird, things are what they really are: an expression of the divine and the perfect. Magical metaphors of everything are created, and the ideals follow after them. A house is not simply a roof over your head, it is a home. A spouse is not only the person with whom you share the duties and education of the children, it is someone you have chosen, a partner in the great journey of life. The concept of honor, of ideals, of the homeland, of the sacred, appears for which many people have been willing to offer their lives. It is the language of the parables of Jesus, the magical stories of the Arabs, Egypt and India and the medieval magical tales of the Zen stories, of mythology, of the Vedas, and of hermeneutics.

At the level of the Hummingbird, we perceive beyond the surface of the conversations and we begin to listen to hidden messages. We read things in the synchronicities that occur with other people. Now this same physical and material world gives us magic and hidden messages. We work with metaphors, and we heal the body by healing the soul. We see paths that will lead us to recover health, and we begin our healing journey. It is not simply performing a ritual without logic, because the concrete logic corresponds to the lower level of the Puma. The level of the Hummingbird is much more powerful and produces changes greater than the Puma. That is why ritualization, psycho-magic, visualization and imagination is more powerful than the simple recitation of positive affirmations, or mental suggestions. During the 60s, Dr. William Kroger, the famous American hypnotherapist realized this, without having understood it correctly. It is the level of the state that I name as the "*twilight states of mind*" or "unbalance states" and many other things that correct the errors of hypnosis and NLP.

We can use many techniques in our lives to develop the perception of the Hummingbird, including meditation, as suggested by Dr. Gerard Encausse himself or Rudolph Steiner or a Zen master, or the "*twilight states of the mind,*" or the development of the relational ability of the mind, of prayer, of music and art. When you want to make sure that your future is going to have a desirable result, you need to visualize it a few times from the perception level of the Hummingbird. If we act from the lower level of the Puma, from the subconscious, we will have to repeat the verbal affirmation, or mental decrees, dozens or maybe hundreds of times to obtain a similar result. There is another way that works, which I have called the "evolutionary therapy," which consists of looking for the reasons at the level of the soul for the different conflicting or problematic conditions in our lives, such as financial, relationship, emotional, physical difficulties, bad luck, and many more. We can also use the Andean Code of "Wisdom,"

IACHEY, creating symbols and representations of the problem through a ritual presented to the lower level of consciousness expecting results from the physical level of matter so that our psyche assumes it is real. In this way, we may make it real; by using a psycho-magical act, we can create a better situation in our life.

At the level of the Hummingbird, the goals that are sought are unlike the level of the Puma. "True goals" are those that cannot be put into a simple concrete "plan of action," as done through common therapies, because of their amplitude, and because it doesn't consider the unknown factors in the equation. These involve the "emerging phenomenon," the participation of the Universe with multiple synchronies impossible to explain, with "implicit learning," changes made in us completely out of consciousness; these I have called "the path of the 10 magical steps of achievement."

At the level of the Hummingbird, the concepts of the "Law of the 3 Forces," "the Evolutionary Triads," and "Law of the Seven," have also been discovered and understood. These are subjects that I have been teaching my students in different trainings, seminars, courses and programs, that have allowed us to understand what happens in the physical world from a very superior level. The goal is to receive answers to very complex situations in life from this level of consciousness, the level of the Hummingbird. At this level, premonitory dreams and instructive dreams and valuable messages for our benefit are produced. At the level of the Hummingbird, Joseph, the father of Jesus, was warned that he should flee to Egypt. Also occurring at this level was Pharaoh's dream of the seven skinny cows and seven fat cows that he could not interpret. And, at this level, Joseph had the dream of the spikes that bowed before him.

The mysterious **Nazca Lines** represent exactly what it is to perceive from different levels of reality. It is a metaphor left there for future generations by the "Guardians of Wisdom" of the Andes. These lines, almost 900 feet long and not more than 1 foot deep, cannot be observed from the ground level - symbolically from the levels of the Serpent and the Puma. They can only be seen when viewed from above, at the levels of the Hummingbird and the Condor. Some have called these mysterious lines "the vision of the gods." Because it is a vision that can only be seen from above, some people think that they were designed by beings from outer space. But the

"Guardians of Wisdom," who handled extremely well metaphorical or relational thinking, thus left an evident metaphor for the coming millennia of the 4 different levels of reality and perception that we have been making known in this book.

It is a lesson written in lines, dug in the ground, noting that certain things cannot be observed or understood from the floor level, from the ground, because they pass - like the Nazca Lines - completely unnoticed or not understood from there. But if we rise to other levels of perception, from the levels of the birds that fly, like the Hummingbird (viewed from the surrounding hills, not very high) or the Condor (vision from the great heights), we can then appreciate and understand them very clearly. To leave no doubt that it was a metaphorical teaching of the different levels of reality and perception they were leaving there, the builders of the Nazca Lines engraved on the ground the drawings of a Hummingbird, a Condor and a Serpent, among the lines.

The true teaching for humanity of the Nazca Lines is that certain problems or situations can be generated at higher levels than the emotional or physical mental reality. That is, on the levels of the psyche (Hummingbird) or the spirit (Condor). And we can only appreciate, understand and solve them, when we rise to the level above the ground. Because from the lower levels - of the concrete, or emotional mind, or of the physical reality itself - it is completely impossible to do so. Transmitting the same teaching of the wise builders of the Nazca Lines - but without metaphors and to be understood by anyone - is one of the objectives of this book.

The level of the Hummingbird is a very powerful level because it is so close to the Condor. But unlike the level of the Condor, where it is not possible to cause any evil, at the level of the Hummingbird, the power of this level can generate evils just like the levels of the Puma and the Serpent. One of them has to do with the level itself because living exclusively on this level of reality can transform you into the world of fantasy and myth, and if the person is too impractical to live a material life, they might not be able to sustain or support themselves in everyday life. The level of the Hummingbird can produce utopias and unreal chimeras, false ideals that later do not agree with the physical reality, along with true "poisoned dreams," that will never work successfully on the material or physical plane.

Thus, at the level of the Hummingbird, multiple utopian and chimerical philosophies may arise, which do not agree with the level of matter, the Serpent, and lead to perdition those who follow them, whether you are an individual, collective, society or organization and whether the group is a religious, economic, philosophical or political movement. In the history of humanity, there have been several examples of these utopias that have led to disasters among groups, collectivities, nations, socialisms, economies and political movements. That´s why the life of a "guardian of knowledge" must always be balanced by the level of the Serpent, or materialism, and always be verified at the level of concrete facts.

Don Joaquin, when teaching me how to weave the energy belts in my "luminous energy sphere," which is a very important ancient Inca drill, pointed out to me that these belts of energy, (which he called "CHUMPIS," pronounced "choompees") are centers of perception of the 4 realities. They should always work in coordination and balance with each other, from the highest reality to the lowest reality. Only in this way did the "Guardians of Wisdom" gain mastery.

Develop the Four Levels in a Balanced Way

You should never underestimate or overestimate anything but live always in the 4 levels simultaneously. You should live in complete balance always and you should practically "review" the drawings of those bands in your "luminous energy sphere" every day, until they become something stable in you. Hence, the extreme importance of developing the 4 levels in a balanced way, because they are fully connected to each other. And for that reason, the priests of the Inca empire who were masters and "Guardians of Wisdom," had a greeting among them that was official for all the citizens of the empire: "You will not be an idler (level of the Serpent), you will not be a liar (level of Puma and Hummingbird), you will not be a thief (level of the Condor that lives in the Ayni and never takes anything what that we have not given something for it)." But other evils can also occur at this level and this evil consists in misdirecting the imagination and faith, and this has also been known by the "keepers of wisdom" for millennia.

At this level the AYNI, or "Sacred Reciprocity" between beings and things, begins to flow more spontaneously. This spiritual concept is more easily understood by the higher mind than by the lower, or concrete mind of the Puma. The AYNI acquires much more sense and begins to be observed as a very valuable way of relating to others. But since this level is still close to that of the Puma, the altruism of the Hummingbird can still be contaminated by the egoism of the Puma. Their broad and powerful capacities can equally be placed unfortunately at the feet of the ego. There is no complete assurance that it will not be like this, and the possibility of being contaminated by the ego ends at the level of the Condor. This level is associated as a door that leads to the divine world, called "HANAK PACHA" by the "Guardians of Wisdom" in the Andes.

Drills at the Level of the Hummingbird

What images do you have more frequently in your "PSIQUIS," or higher mind?

If your imagination that is held in your mind's eye is what you want to see, such as a beautiful body, youthfulness, and health, or in your personal life, like prosperity, good relationships with others, or love, then keep on supporting it and sheltering them constantly until they become a reality. But if they are not, completely refrain from them, don't allow your powerful imagination or image-building psyche to build a poor house and continually hold that image in your mind. Eventually you will be attracted to that poor house and live as miserably as if you were already there. *Many people have reached premature old age, disability or death because they have been controlled by their imagination and their faith has unconsciously made them a reality*, instead of being owners of it and controlling it efficiently.

Exercise 1

The Mirror

Look at yourself in a mirror and begin to imagine that your physical body disappears. Let your body and energetic vital manifestation of your being, at the level of the Serpent, disappear. Now, let the emotional and mental aspect of your being, disappear. Let all the thoughts of the concrete world and the emotions experienced in your life, at the level of the Cougar, disappear. Now, only you remain in front of the mirror, with your nakedness beheld in your mind's eye and your psyche at the highest level, at the level of Hummingbird, and with your Divine Soul.

When you achieve this experience, talk to your psyche, giving it powerful messages or powerful images. Imprint all your achievements there; state, or imagine, what you want to obtain in life, and in relationship to your own person, as if they were already a reality. You will be entering powerful codes into your "luminous energy sphere" that will change everything.

But I give you an *important warning* here: since this level is still close to that of the Puma, **the altruism of the Hummingbird can still be contaminated by the egoism of the Puma**. Therefore, the warning I am making here is that you must be extremely careful when practicing this drill, like all others at this level; make sure you are only guided by the principle of AYNI for the good of yourself and of others. Never allow the broad and powerful capabilities at this level to be placed at the foot of your little ego, or to harm other beings in the least. The AYNI works like a boomerang, if you harm others, then you will be the first one to be injured; if you benefit others, the beneficiary will also be you.

Exercise 2

Social Interaction

Start doing the same thing with other people you see, with whom you are talking, or who you see on the street, in a restaurant, etc. Perform the above Exercise until you have the feeling that you can communicate with their psyche. Remember again to always live under the AYNI, or the "Sacred Reciprocity" in each Exercise and with everything that surrounds you. If you harm others, the first harmed will be you. If you benefit others, the beneficiary will also be you. It is the main teaching of the Andes.

Exercise 3

Creating the "Twilight State"
of the mind

There are endless ways to produce this powerful state of mind, that I discovered years ago, and in daily life it often occurs spontaneously. The important thing here is to learn to create it consciously when you want to create it and not just as a state created by chance. I will offer you three different ways to create it, choose the one you like the most or is the most friendly and simple for you.

Practice this Exercise once a day, in a quiet place, and hopefully silent, where nobody will interrupt you. When you have completed this practice time, you can enter and exit the state with great ease. The *unbalance or twilight state is used for different purposes*, according to the polarity:

Active use of the state: To produce changes and aids or improvements in any department of the subconscious, like in the cognitive, emotional or organic states, in transformations and reparative processes or generative changes. It can be used in a busy environment.

Passive, receptive use of the state: To develop inspiration, creativity or genius. It is recommended only in quiet places and in a place where there are no other people. It is further explained in Exercise 4, below.

Exercise 4 (A-C)

First Method to Produce "Twilight State" (For Visual People)

4A.   Through a visual hallucination

Look at a wall, or door or object, and whatever the color of that wall, door or object is, with open eyes, imagine it taking on a different color. For example, if it is white, then imagine it turning red, blue or green in your mind. Make it the one you want. Once this is happening, with your imagination, having allowed this color to change, you are already in the "twilight state of the mind." Close your eyes and keep seeing that imaginary color. You can do it by looking at a person's eyes and imagining that they change to another color. Now, only deepen this state using the general deepening dynamics that appears after the "Third Method" in this series of Exercises. While what you are seeing continues with this new imaginary color, eventually everything will end, and you will not pay attention to it anymore.

Second Method of Producing the "Twilight State" (Hearing People)

4B. Through an auditory hallucination

Allow your imagination to hear a bell or any other imaginary sound like the wind, a song, melody or a musical instrument. While in your mind, you imaginatively allow that sound to grow and continue. You are already in the "twilight state of the mind." Now, only deepen the state using the general deepening dynamics. While the sound will continue in the background until everything ends, you will not pay attention to it.

Third Method to Produce "Twilight State" (Kinesthetic People)

4C.   Through a kinesthetic hallucination

Sitting on a chair or lying on a bed, put your hands and arms on your legs. Allow your imagination to make you feel that a very heavy object (for example a sack of flour or several of them on top of each other) falls on one of your hands and arms. The weight of these bags, in your imagination, is so heavy that it traps and completely immobilizes that arm and hand. Allow your imagination to be so real that it is impossible for you to lift your arms or hands when you try. When this is happening, you are already in the "twilight state of the mind." Now, only deepen the state using the deepening dynamics. While the feeling of weight on your arm will be there all the time, you will not pay attention to it.

Put your attention inward, on your mind. There you will see all the letters of the alphabet that you learned when you were a child - from

A to Z - and from which you read, write and speak. Imagine now that an imaginary vacuum machine enters your mind and begins to suck and remove those letters from your mind, one by one. While the letters are going out through the tube of that vacuum machine, it will also take with them the unnecessary thoughts, and any worries that we do not need at this particular time. Give permission for this to happen… just imagine this happening without making any effort other than giving permission for this to happen.

Carefully watch, listen and feel in your mind, how the letters leave one by one. Each of them is going through the tube of the vacuum cleaner and disintegrating within it. As this happens you go into a very pleasant, deep and very pleasant, mental rest; a special void or quiet place, as the letters are leaving through the tube and disintegrating there. Let it go to the last of the letters and, in that instant, your mind enters that deep, pleasant and healing rest.

In that moment, when the last one was gone, even if you wanted to remember some of those letters, it will not be possible for you. Because you have given them full permission to leave your mind. When you finish the drill, they will return without any problem, when this

Exercise is over; but until that moment, they will not be in your mind, and you will not be able to bring them around until you turn off the vacuum cleaner. Give mental permission for this to happen. Once the last letter has gone, allow the vacuum cleaner to continue to suck and maintain a vacuum in your mind, all the time, just in case a naughty thought or desire wants to return, which will not be allowed, because it will be immediately absorbed again by the vacuum cleaner. The vacuum cleaner will continue to guard your thoughts, with your permission, the entire time you are in this state. When you're completely in the vacuum, and the vacuum cleaner is there maintaining the vacuum in your mind, continue with whatever you are trying to achieve, while in this "twilight state of the mind." You will be fully aware and more aware than ever in this pleasant emptiness.

Exercise 5. (A-E)

Active Use of the Twilight State to Exercise Direct Action on the Physical Body – Level of the Serpent

Example 5A.   To Stop Allergies and the possibility of anaphylactic shock

The "twilight state of the mind" is induced using any of the three dynamics and deepened by the "deepening dynamics." Then, the following words are delivered as suggestions:

"All danger has gone away and there was no danger, that's why all the inflammation stops now, completely now, the inflammation disappears because there is no danger, there was never any danger, it was a falsity. Stop filtering fluid, that's why all the inflammation stops now, completely now, everything returns to normal because there is no danger, there was never any danger, it was a falsity, everything returns to normal!

And these suggestive words continue to be offered for about 5 minutes. Then all this must be repeated every half hour until the danger is completely over or the allergy disappears. In my personal experience with 6 daily applications for two or three days, any allergic symptoms are stopped only using these words in the "twilight state of the mind."

Example 5B.   To Stop Headache

The "twilight state of the mind" is induced and deepened. The following words are delivered:

*"The pain fades and disappears completely, it vanishes, it goes
away; the pain fades and disappears completely, it vanishes, it goes away".*

This is repeated for about 5 minutes, 2 or 3 times until the pain completely disappears

Example 5C.   To Adjust the Levels of Glucose in the Blood

The "twilight state of the mind" is induced and deepened. The following words are delivered:

"Now the blood glucose level is adjusted to a normal, healthy lower

level, the glucose level falls to an ideal level and you get a good and optimal health condition, now that high glucose level is corrected. This adjustment is being done NOW until everything is normalized in the blood, your body will continue to do this even when you open your eyes, and each time you pass through a doorway the glucose level will be sure to be at its normal level in your blood."

This is repeated for about 5 minutes, 2 or 3 times.

Example 5D.   To Decrease Blood Pressure

The twilight state of the mind is induced and deepened. The following words are delivered:

"The level of pressure exerted by the blood on the wall of the arteries is now adjusted, blood pressure falls to normal levels, the force exerted by the blood on the arteries is reduced, the internal mechanisms do their work so that blood pressure level is corrected to levels that are beneficial. Take the necessary time for this adjustment until everything is normalized in the pressure

that the blood exerts on the walls of the arteries. Even when you open your eyes, and every time you pass through a doorway, blood pressure will be sure to be at its normal level."

This is repeated for about 5 minutes, 2 or 3 times until blood pressure has normalized.

Example 5E.   Secretion of an Abundant Number of Endorphins in the Body

The "twilight state" is induced and deepened. The following words are delivered:

"An enormous quantity of endorphins are entering your bloodstream right now, these are the chemical substances that your own body manufactures, and which provide inner well-being and a state of happiness. Your body right now manufactures these happiness drugs in enormous quantities and makes them enter the blood, secreting large amounts inside you, filling the blood and traveling to each cell of your body, making you feel extraordinarily well and happy. Allow this to happen right now. Your body is becoming so full of them

that you cannot believe how good you begin to feel. These endorphins are filling your body in huge quantities right now, and all these happiness drugs circulate throughout your body all day long. This will not end when you open your eyes. All day long, even when you leave this state, you will be full of these substances feeling amazing and fantastic like never before."

This is repeated for about 5 minutes.

Exercise 6

Passive or Receptive
Use of the Twilight State

"Sitting in Silence"
Dr. Elmer Gates,
of Chevy Chase, Maryland

It is well known that through the process of cultivating and using the creative faculty, the inspirational inventor, Dr. Elmer R. Gates, created more than 200 useful patents in the United States. For anyone who feels interested in attaining the status of genius, in whose category Dr. Gates belonged, his method is significant and fascinating at the same time. In his laboratory, he had what he called his "personal communication room." It was a noise-proof room and arranged in such a way that every flash of light could be eliminated. It was equipped with a small table on which he always had a notebook. In front of the table, on the wall, there was a panel of electrical switches that controlled the lights. When Dr. Gates wanted to use the thought force that was available to him through the "twilight state" of his mind, he would enter the room, sit at the table, turn off the lights, and concentrate on the known factors of the invention. There he remained in that position until the ideas began to appear in his mind, in connection with the unknown factors of the invention. Once the ideas came to his mind, they came so quickly that he was forced to write right away. When the thoughts stopped flowing, and he examined the notes he had taken, he discovered that he had a meticulous description of principles, unparalleled among all those known to the scientific world. In addition, the answer to his problem was intelligently presented in these notes.

The faculty of solving problems with the logical mind, many times turns out to be defective, because it is guided, in good measure, only by one's accumulated knowledge and experience, and not all the knowledge one has is accurate or correct. The ideas received by the "twilight stage of the mind" are much more consistent, for the simple reason that they come from sources more reliable than those obtained by the reasoning faculty of the ordinary mind, such as from indiscriminate books read, offhand suggestions from others, etc.

So, if you want to have inspirations, sit in silence like Dr. Gates, as many others did before and after him. Enter the "twilight state of the mind," using some of the methods already given in this book and pose your question in concrete terms. The answer will come. If not at that moment, in a similar one, or when you are somewhere else, or reading a book, or doing something else, or in a dream; the answer could even be brought by a friend when talking to you.

Exercise 7

Methods for Developing Intuition Daily

7A. Each time you want to know the time of day, stop for a moment before looking at the time, enter a brief twilight state for just a few seconds and focus on the question: What is the exact time? The answer can come as an image with numbers, or as a feeling of knowing the time, or a phrase that tells the time inside the mind. You must capture the first impression that arrives and do not allow a second, third or fourth impression to modify it. Then look at the watch to see if your intuition has been correct.

Remember to check the accuracy not only from *your* watch, but also from others, because your watch may be ahead or behind the actual time. The second, third or fourth impression is always the result of your analytical mind, which is not intuitive; these impressions must always be rejected. From the education you have received all your life, you try to usurp the first one, which is the only one that is legitimate. At the beginning of these Exercises, there will occur many of these first impressions that are wrong, because the intuitive faculty is just exercising consciously, and the correct answers will not yet be fully captured by you until you acquire more practice. As you have been accustomed to using ONLY your concrete mind, in the beginning it will be the analytical mind also that will make the first impression. But, with the repetitions of these Exercises, you will achieve success in this training. And this will improve even more as you become more and more expert in twilight thinking. *The essential practice that you must acquire is to leave your concrete mind, level of the Puma, completely aside. This will take some time and constant Exercise. It is the great stopping stone, in the path of this training, that we must learn to overcome.*

7B. Each time our phone rings or vibrates, instead of answering immediately, enter a very brief twilight state for just a few seconds and ask yourself: "Who is calling?" And then, "Why is he calling me?" Remember that the first impression that arrives, is the one that you must always accept, even if it is a strange response to your mind. Remember that intuition always enters unknown terrain. Doing this will prevent you from establishing the habit of listening to the second, third or fourth impression. If during the first 20 or more times your answers are wrong, you should not be discouraged, but continue with the practice until you get more and more right guesses or intuitive answers.

Remember that the essential practice that you must acquire through these Exercises is to learn to "deprogram," and thus learn, step by step, to leave your analytical and logical mind completely aside. This will take some time, and constant practice, because it's been years that you've done the opposite in your life. Intuition already exists in you and is fully active in the "higher pole of your being," because you are a human. It is your natural inheritance. The aim of these Exercises is not so much to develop it, because it already exists and is active, but to "de-program" and prevent the analytical logical-mind, and rational mind, from blocking it and not letting it work.

7C. You must also do the same with each message that arrives to your cell phone, or email, even with the physical mail that can reach you. Before reading it, or opening the message, or the envelope, enter a very brief twilight state, for just a few seconds, and ask yourself: "Who sent me this message?" and

"What content does it have?"

7D. We can also enter during the day into a very brief twilight state, for just a few seconds, and ask ourselves certain questions that we do not know within the concrete mind and wait for the answer in silence. The intuitive skills that will be developed to receive knowledge with these Exercises will be instantaneous. There will be a moment when, before completing the question, you will receive the answer from a message or a phone call, etc. All these Exercises are to allow the mind to stop depending on the habit of using just reason, and the usual analysis at the Puma level that we have accepted so far without any objection and get used to letting the intuition begin to participate in the process and start replacing it. The difficulty you may encounter in these Exercises is due exclusively to the coordinated social programming that exists against intuition. All the training of a "civilized" human being conspires against intuition, which is one of the most desirable and extraordinary capacities or functions of our being.

Our educational achievements and mental developments have been programmed at the higher levels of all education, including colleges and universities, which have conspired against intuition. The measurements of "aptitudes," that are made on people to be accepted into a college or university, is based on tests that measure the capacity of reasoning, analysis and logic; including memory capacity and the speed of learning that a person has in the use of these capacities. With this system of measuring educational aptitude, the "intelligence" or "potential" of a human being is measured unfairly for his intellectual capacity or supposed "disability." For this reason, the beginning of these Exercises could seem difficult, and you may make many mistakes at first, because your logical, rational and analytical mind will be blocking your intuition, that already exists, and will not let it work. This social conspiracy must be unlearned.

Intuition is the highest quality of the human mind, and it is latent in the majority of people. This ability is completely trainable in most people and when it is developed, it will become the highest kind of clairvoyance. It will then consist of an effortless, instantaneous activity of facts, principles, events and uncanniness. The way to develop it is simple: *when an intuitive sensation manifests itself in you, test its veracity immediately*. In a short time with this Exercise, it will become clearer and more accurate, stronger, fuller and more frequent.

Exercise 8
Examples A-H

8A. Replace the answers and reflex ideas that come only from the memory at the level of the Puma, with one's reasoned or experienced ideas from the level of the Hummingbird, which are measured and thoughtful responses. The worst enemy is the floating mass of thoughtful ideas, that come to us from the books that we have read or studied, social media, news media etc., which are presented to our reasoning mind constantly. The memory, at the level of the Puma, must always be subject to the active intelligence of the psyche from the level of the Hummingbird.

8B. Arguments with other people should be completely avoided. By wounding their convictions, all we get in return is the incitement of their self-love and thus we convert the semi-convinced into an irreducible enemy of the ideas we propose. I advise to keep quiet whenever we see an ardent discussion on a subject, let's avoid it completely. We must teach, say what we think, but we must respect ourselves enough to never enter the field of discussions in which the intellectual faculties of the concrete mind, focused on the level of the Serpent or Puma, are used so uselessly.

8C. Through development of analog or relational thinking, through analogical thinking, gigantic truths are obtained behind the physical and external forms in everyday life. It is good to learn to see with the intelligence from the psychic being, the human soul or higher mind, and not only "look" at these automatic and unconscious acts, but also at the facts that are presented to us daily. Stop looking from the level of the Serpent. It is important to know how to find the IDEA that hides behind everyday events or the physical world. This is the level of the Hummingbird. When we have a problem, we learn to detect why it originated, rise above the problem and look to nature for something that allows us to solve it. All this is an experience of the level of the Hummingbird. It is important to look for relationships that link different ideas, and this is only possible through analogies or relational thinking. One should search within oneself, and not out of books, for the analogies of natural things. This has been the science of shamans, and of wild men, who in this way have been able to discover the healing properties of certain herbs or stones; and also, of the great inventors like Tesla and Einstein and of the simple men, who by means of analogies, came to understand great laws or hidden principles.

8D. Do not accept any physical sensation without avoiding the subconscious reaction of pleasure or dislike that it provokes. This must be a constant Exercise that also helps us to develop the active faculty of the Will efficiently, also, from the level of the Hummingbird.

8E. You are recommended to practice the intense and prolonged contemplation of works of art, as well as the observation of the works of nature, like a stone, a flower, or a tree. If one lives in a big city and has the opportunity to visit important museums, this is highly recommended. These contemplations, just as with natural works, must be done on the days and within the hours when there are not many people; doing so in moments in which there is as much silence as possible. This method applies, as well, to the works of nature, and requires several sessions of meditation on a single work of art. Let the mind, without prejudice and without recourse to memory, receive the ideas that emanate from the painting or sculpture.

8F. We can also do this with great literary works, such as the poems of Homer, the Bible, the works of Shakespeare, the Upanishads of India, or the books of Sri Aurobindo. It is recommended that you use only masterpieces universally recognized for the inspiration of passive ideas. You must have a pencil and paper to write down the ideas suggested by that work.

8G. Following the instructions of Pythagoras, it is beneficial at night before falling asleep, to review everything that happened during the day. From the last moment of the day, to the beginning of the day (like an upside-down movie), review how you acted, noticing if anything was done in a wrong movement. Retain this experience in your memory, especially if it was wrong, in order not to make another mistake.

8H. It is advisable, in the mornings, when getting up, to wrap oneself completely with a blanket of natural wool, including the head, and to remain this way in the bed, focusing your thoughts on the tasks that will be realized that day. This Exercise should be practiced for 5-10 minutes, six times a week. While doing this, your breathing must be slow and deep; after a while, this procedure will produce a great physical well-being from the level of the Hummingbird.

Dr. Rod Fuentes with the young Quero,
Julio Mallki.

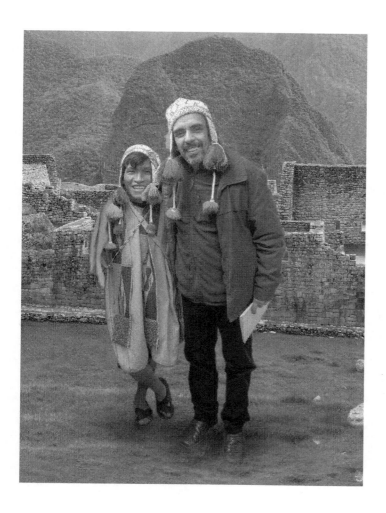

CHAPTER TWELVE

Other Experiences at the Hummingbird Level

Differences between logical thought, lower mind, and intuition of the higher mind at the level of the Hummingbird

I was studying in the second year of Dentistry at the School of Medicine of the University of Chile. At that time, I lived in a very cold place and in an area far from the center of the city of Santiago. One day I woke up early in the morning, at my appointed time for breakfast and then walked to the University. During my walk, I felt a very sharp pain in the instep of my right foot and noticed that I had a very reddened area the size of a small coin. In the center of that reddened area there was a blister the size of just the tip of a pencil, which was the cause of my pain. At that instant I imagined that an insect had bitten me. I thought that possibly a spider had entered my bed and bitten me while I slept. The house spiders in Chile are very dangerous, so I immediately decided, before going to class, that I would go to the medical service for the students at the

University to be treated. When the doctor arrived, I told him about my fears of being stung by a corner spider.

The doctor looked at the blister, but he did not know what it was, and I did not really know if I had been bitten by a spider or not. He was so intrigued that he summoned an entire board of medical specialists and experts, next to me. They soon formed a tight circle around my right foot, with their faces almost glued to my foot looking intrigued and giving their opinion. One said that it looked like a spider bite and that it should not be ruled out. Another said that it was probably a strange new virus that was affecting young people my age, while the others gave other explanations.

Suddenly, I saw that above this circle of doctors, was the shy head of a general doctor, who had not been called but happened to casually be there. Perhaps he was intrigued by the commotion and poked his head into the circle of doctors. While others gave their specialized opinions, he simply said, "It looks like a burn." The others looked back at him with scorn and disdain and continued to completely ignore the doctor who withdrew in silence. When I heard about the burn, I immediately remembered that the night before had been a very cold night, especially in the area where I lived, and I had used a bag of water to warm my feet. I had gone to bed extremely tired and the bag of water had leaked and burned my skin. Of course, I kept silent for fear of being insulted by the group of "scholars," specialists and expert doctors, who had been summoned. I was afraid to interrupt them from their ultra-specialized visions with something as trivial and innocuous as a small burn caused only by hot water bag that had leaked a drop of water over my foot.

The intuition of the less specialized doctor was the only true one and surpassed all the scholarly and ultra-specialized opinions of others. That is the great difference between intuition and "erudition" and logic of the concrete mind, the level of the Puma. The latter is merely the result of the constant use of memory, study, logic and reason, and the conditioning that many times this imposes on our mind and life. Instead of getting closer to the truth, you can completely distance yourself from it. Today, doctors rely on an enormous number of medical tests that intuitive doctors of the past did not need and most of the times they had more certainty in their diagnoses.

The Teachings of Paracelsus, XV Century Physician and Father of Pharmacology

Paracelsus called the diseases caused by the psyche or human soul, which put into action faith and imagination at the Hummingbird level, "invisible diseases." He pointed out that faith and imagination can be the cause of illness and that this is a misuse of faith and the imagination in us. "Faith can take responsibility for all kinds of diseases." He was a doctor who made true miracles with his patients, and he could, with his power of faith, heal or kill his patients; in the same way as physically killing, by administering a healing remedy or a deadly poison like arsenic. For Paracelsus, both were the same.

According to his own words: "Faith works in us like an artisan, who, after forging a knife, can wound another person with it or use it to cut the meat on his plate of food." He pointed out that the Gospels gives a brief exposition of the strength and power of the faith, expressing the following phrase: "If your Faith were only the size of a mustard seed and you said with the strength of that Faith: Mountain, throw yourself into the sea, the mountain would disappear into the waters." But according to his writings, the psyche, moved by his capacities of faith and imagination, not only produce diseases, but all kinds of problems: economic, of relationships between people, accidents, what is called "bad luck" and many other things. *"For with true faith, we can heal a sick body or soul. Carrying that faith within us, we will believe that everything can be possible. In virtue of our faith, we can get sick by it and by it we can heal ourselves."* The great American thinker Prentice Mulford stated that: "If you are sick and you do not cure your problem, it is not that you DO NOT have faith in healing, but you have more faith in the disease." At the level of the Hummingbird or human psyche, much good can be created and much harm can be done equally.

"Imagination not only kills in times of epidemics, but also in times of war. In the sieges of the cities, in the skirmishes, there are soldiers who have not had more than their imagination to have been hit by bullets. Indeed, the one who trembles, the one who flees, the one who is frightened by each detonation, who is constantly afraid of being hit by bullets, is often hit and wounded many more times than the daring intrepid ones, who fear nothing and remain full of hope. The latter are the ones who do not die, survive and take the cities, the fortresses, the land.s" -Paracelsus

A doctor who wrongly decrees a prognosis of a disease as "terminal" or a disease diagnoses as "incurable" even when the disease does not exist, the decree that the doctor gives adds all the potential that can kill a person. In the investigations that he made at the Faculty of Medicine of the University of California, the researcher Norman Simmons determined that of the hundreds of patients who had recovered from cancer, the patients had followed very diverse treatments. Some had followed the traditional medical therapies of chemotherapy or radiotherapy while others used natural therapy, Chinese medicine therapy, Reiki, Biomagnetism, etc. But, when analyzing what it was that had worked with them, and not with those who died, they found that the only thing common among all of them was "the confidence and faith of the person in the treatment they were following."

Sometimes an effect on the physical level can occur completely unconsciously from the level of the Hummingbird, as it happened to someone very close to me. As a teenager he was very interested in a small and unattractive mole that a classmate had on his right leg near the knee. A few months later, an almost identical one appeared on his right leg but a little lower than the one his partner had on her leg.

Mortal Use of the Psyche and Imagination

This is a real-life example about the imagination and misdirected faith, at the psychic or Hummingbird level, which happened to a close relative of the author, as it was transmitted in our family stories.

A young friend of the author's family who was full of opportunities and talents had a fascination for death. At every party to which he was invited, even when he was the most cheerful, he sang poems to death, which he called "dear and beautiful friend," and made a constant public display of this macabre fascination. At the age of 35 he went to visit relatives who had a mill. When crossing over a pulley at those old mills, which was in operation, his scarf and coat were entangled in the pulley and despite all the efforts he made, he could not escape the terrible force that exerted from the machine on his body. Many ran to stop the machine, others to cut the electricity supply that drove the electric mill, but it was too late. His life had a horrible end, giving a frightful spectacle to all who were present. When he died, he was again the center of attention, as he had been before at each party. This time he joined in an obvious and definitive way with his "dear and beautiful friend."

The Great Power for the Good at the Hummingbird Level

"Thoughts floating in the air are like beings struggling to achieve life, seeking to materialize in the physical world." - Anonymous.

With the activity at the level of the human soul, higher mind or "psyche," many forces develop, among them the greatest of all forces, that of thought. When accompanied by imagination and faith, thought is one of the greatest manifestations of Universal energy. He who understands the use of this energy can do practically whatever he wants. Not only is the body of a person being subject to the domain of the mind, but also the environment, such as "luck," fate and circumstances. From here arises the convenience of replacing negative thoughts and imaginations with positive ones. The attitude and thoughts "I want, and I am capable," if at the same time, are full of the fuel of imagination and faith (without these it will not work well) and leads us towards an achievement and success that seems miraculous to another person placed on the plane, "I cannot do it. "

"The soldier who aspires to a high fortune, must have before the eyes of his imagination Julius Caesar, or one of the famous warriors among the Romans. If he knows how to properly use his imagination, if he is fully determined to resist until the end, if he is enlightened in wars, he will reach the highest honors. Many ignore how imagination and faith can lead to honors and riches. Some could object that they have come to the honors thanks to luck or their hard work. I testify that the imagination commands all things and that faith, exalts everything ..." - Paracelsus.

Healing Disease Example of Healing from the Hummingbird Level of the Psyche (Higher Mind)

"Your Faith has healed you…"
- Matthew 10: 46-52

At the house of a friend, a maid provided domestic services to his family. She had a 12-year-old daughter, who came with her mother to his home, several times a week. This little girl was very pretty but was affected by several warts on different parts of her body including the arms, hands, legs and back. There were so many warts that the dermatologists, who had seen her, had not been able to provide a good solution in her case. My friend's father, who had a great curiosity about the "powers of the mind," had read somewhere, probably Paracelsus, that if a doctor produced an intense mental-emotional impact on his patient, he could produce amazing cures. As there was nothing to lose, he decided to put this theory to the test. One day he approached the girl and her mother and told them that he had a "secret" that had been communicated to him many years ago as "infallible" to relieve the girl of her problems; but they should not discuss it with anyone.

This secret was about waiting for the Full Moon in the countryside, in front of a rock. Exactly at midnight, she had to make 21 turns around the rock, without stopping, fixing her eyes on the stars, the moon or the sky. She was instructed to shout, "heaven take away these warts." But she should not stop at any moment or stop looking at the sky during the 21 rounds. This story had been invented by my friend's father; nobody had ever communicated it to him as a "secret." The mother looked for a place in the countryside where there would be a rock and there were some relatives that had a farm that met the conditions. They made the preparations and waited until the arrival of the Full Moon. They proceeded exactly as they had been told, the mother was counting the turns while the girl just repeated the mysterious words and did not stop looking at the sky. Having done this, they went to sleep. After 7 days all the warts had disappeared from the girl's body.

Power of Imagination and Faith in a Case of Terminal Cancer

This is a tragic story that comes from the 1950s. These events show the miraculous powers of the human psyche, at the

Hummingbird level, and how healing this level can be if triggered with the correct frame and mental attitude. This is the story of Mr. Wright, a fictitious name out of respect for his family, according to one of the doctors who treated his case in a report by Dr. Philip West. Mr. Wright had lymphatic cancer, or lymphosarcoma, in an advanced degree. He had tumors in the neck, armpits, groin and abdomen. He was about to die, and the doctors could only administer analgesics. There was no hope.

Mr. Wright had illusions that he would soon discover a remedy for this disease. When he learned of the drug, Krebiozen, that would be tested in the hospital where he was, he asked to have it administered to him. He was accepted, even though he should not have taken it because the trial was to be done only on patients with a prognosis of survival of at least three months of life; and he was dying. He received three injections in total.

Wright had been confined to bed rest for weeks, but two days after the first injection he was walking through the hospital ward and talking to the nurses. The tumors were reduced to half their previous size. Ten days later he was discharged. Prior to the experimental drug, he had to wear a respirator, but two weeks later, he piloted his private plane at an altitude of 12,000 feet. None of the other patients to whom the drug was administered experienced the slightest improvement. The drug was completely innocuous.

When Mr. Wright knew this, he became very depressed, and after two months of perfect health, he relapsed to his previous state. The tumors returned and grew larger and again he was on the verge of death. The doctor who treated him gave him new hope. The drug had failed because it deteriorated in storage, but it was predicted that the next day there would come a new batch of double power. This was not true, but the patient regained hope with such news. He was given the first injection of the "new double potency preparation" but, only water was injected. This time the patient recovered more quickly than before. He soon returned to normal life and flew back in his private plane with full health.

After 2 months, the press announced that the AMA (American Medical Association) had declared the drug completely ineffective for cancer. Days after the news, the patient was again admitted to the hospital in serious condition. The tumors reappeared, and Mr. Wright died two days later.

Even though he passed away, he leaves us with an important legacy. Those powerful results where the tumors dissolved, and the return to a healthy life, demonstrate the power of the human psyche, the higher mind, that set-in motion positive imagination and faith. This is the power at the level of the Hummingbird. And when the right conditions are present, the mind triggers an inner healing and magical ability, where the most amazing and surprising results can appear. This potential healer, at the level of the Hummingbird, the human psyche, resides within each one of us. The only challenge is to know how to trigger it. This is what I am explaining in this book, as was taught to me by the "Guardians of Wisdom," in the Andean Mountains.

Acting on Ourselves at the Hummingbird Level

Whoever wants to succeed must always, with his desire and imagination - live, move, think and act as if he had already achieved that success - this attitude is the magnetic force that makes realization possible. The "guardians of knowledge," who we think so highly about, and value so much, are without ego or pride. When they are forced to temporarily occupy what the world calls a humble place; they embrace it as though it were their legitimate sphere.

The "guardians of knowledge" are the ones who live the most in their thoughts, since thought is the power that brings to them the corresponding material part that they are looking for. If they would mentally be challenged in the presence of the strength or talents of others, or because of the sumptuousness in which others live, there could be created a kind of envious humiliation. Then the lower vibrations that impact the realm of the human soul, the Hummingbird, caused by such thoughts and feelings, could immediately put many obstacles in their paths that would be very difficult for them to overcome. This is well known to the "guardians of knowledge," and is the reason why they learned to think always with optimism and hope, as if the excellent things that the world has to offer were already theirs.

Years ago, I reactivated a group of people, founded almost a century ago in Santiago, Chile, called "*The Circle.*" It is based on learning to activate the capacities, and operate efficiently at the Hummingbird level, to obtain results and advances in any of the different areas that make up our life. "The Circle" is based on the principle that just as our physical bodies, after being duly trained, can become highly developed, thereby obtaining extraordinary physical abilities in the physical world with amazing results; the same is possible for the lesser-known and obvious human soul skills and abilities, at the reality level of the Hummingbird.

"Even when you drink water from an old jug, at the level of the Serpent, IMAGINE THAT YOU DRINK FROM A SILVER CUP."

"Even if your shoes are pierced, in your mind VISUALIZE that you wear new and luxurious shoes".

"Even if your clothes are old and cheap, imagine that you wear the most beautiful, fine and elegant of the costumes."

"The human being who is on the true path to success, not only knows and fully trusts that he is capable of achieving his goal, but at the same time forces his mental Image to materialize through his actions."

"He acts as if he has already achieved his goal." **El Círculo** *– by Rod Fuentes.*

CHAPTER THIRTEEN

Perceptions from the Spiritual Level of the Condor

The Language of Living Energy

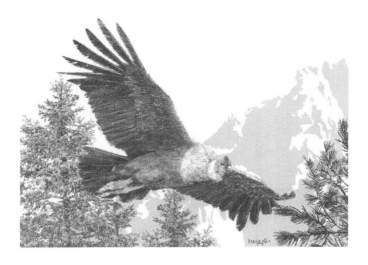

Like the Hummingbird, the Condor also flies, but much higher. Therefore, it moves further away than the Hummingbird from the lower levels of animals that move at ground level, like the Serpent and the Puma. The level of the Hummingbird was high, but the Condor is the highest of all levels of human perception. When we observe something on this level, we see God experiencing himself in the form of an event or person. When the Condor flies over a valley, it can see everything with its peripheral vision - the trees, the mountains, the river, the horizon, even the curvature of the Earth, because the Condor has its eyes at its sides, which gives it an extremely wide field of view. It therefore has the capacity to see globally but can also observe small units or things at a distance; this is a quality of the Spirit at this level.

At the level of the Condor, reality is 99% consciousness and 1% matter. For this reason, one of the characteristics at the level of the Condor is the "timelessness and non-existence of distance or space," because time and space are determining characteristics at the physical level; that is, the level of the Serpent, which is very far from this level. The main communication is that of energy exchange. The brain structure associated with this level is the prefrontal cortex, which is a structure involved in the planning of cognitively complex behaviors. When it is damaged in an adult, it makes him irritable, impatient and with high deficits of social and interpersonal relationship. The prefrontal cortex develops slowly until adulthood, which could explain, at least in part, why young people have less development of it and greater tendency to participate in risky activities and perform less rational choices in favor of impulsive decisions.

At the level of the Condor, everything is understood as constant exchanges of energy, though, in different manifestations. It is displayed as feelings or acts, between people, between beings, and between all things and is the Spirit feeding the Spirit. It is the level of kindness, of gentleness, of pure altruism, of the noblest feelings, and of faith, and constant hope, and of unity in everything without separations.

In the movie "Pocahontas", by Disney, she explains to the Englishman John Smith, the *interconnected energy* of the Universe, in the following way:

"The rainstorm and the river are my brothers... *And we are all connected to each other in a circle,* in a hoop that never ends."

What she is describing to the Englishman, who lives on the level of the Serpent, is literally an energetic description from the level of the Condor. At this level we begin to feel and manifest the conditions of altruism. The "golden rule" which was attributed to Jesus, was taught by all the great guides of humanity. The universal principles, the Andean codes, that are described in this book, all emerged from this level of perception and existence. At this level, the energy is expressed through the message: "Love others as yourself," which is presented by Hermes, Krishna, Buddha, Jesus, and Pachacuti in the Andes. All of them had a full perception from the highest level of the Condor. Here, we begin to dissolve the physical separation and time element from people and things and begin to observe ourselves together as parts of a single being, with the powerful vision of the Condor. By helping another, I help myself. When I treat another with kindness, I do it also to myself. The good of others, along with their happiness, makes me happy. Everything returns to me. Here the energetic relations with the whole Universe are expressed, which the Andean codes call AYNI, the "Sacred Reciprocity" of God in everything. This was the law given to the human beings in the Andes.

The AYNI, "Sacred Reciprocity" or "Andean Gratitude," is the very essence of this level. At this level it would be impossible to understand our existence without AYNI. At the level of the Condor, I no longer think only of myself, as I did at the level of the Serpent or Puma, where the concepts of space and separation temporally exists, and individuality and selfishness govern. Now I think of the welfare of all, because everyone's welfare is also mine. Here the separatism, the individuality, the competition of the Puma comes to an end, and there appears the unity, the common good, the support for the weakest, and the cooperation among all. At this level it is understood that we are all linked as one unit, and that there is no real separation between beings and things. We understand that if there is someone trapped in the lower levels and suffering in some way, we cannot be completely free or happy either.

Physical and mental barriers begin to dissolve when the individual souls of all people begin to recognize their unity at this level, their brotherhood. Here - time, matter, space and distance - disappear as physical barriers. We perceive ourselves as connected by energy ties or "segues," or filaments of light to each other and through them we are united to distant places, although separated by thousands of miles, or even by time; even with those who live in another time or are separated by death. Because at this level we become aware of the timelessness and lack of distance or space. We are thus equally united, energetically, and connected to the stars. We are connected to all beings, animals, trees, stones, rivers, the animate and inanimate things. And we can establish mental and spiritual connections with a star that can be transformed into our guide. Or we can connect with the Earth, or with a spiritual being that has its connection with the physical world through a sacred mountain.

At this level we explain the Andean code Kawsay, or "Existence," where a stone can represent our existence, or can be intentionally transformed by you into a clone of yourself; or a sheet of paper can represent a part of you as your problems, or doubts, or confusions, etc. When you ask a "guardian of knowledge" of the Andes who he is, he will tell you from this level: "I am the snowy peaks, I am the sea, the lake, the Condor, the rock, the valley, I am all of them." From the level of the Puma, he will see himself as a person with a history, with determined parents, but from the level of the Condor, he knows that God is disguised as a particular being. A "guardian of wisdom" resides on the heights of the Condor. When we face a difficulty, the closer we get to the level of the Divine Soul (Spirit or Atman), the less energy we will need to change things.

In the lower levels of the animals that move on the Earth, we can try to find a way to avoid war. But, at the level of the Condor, we can become peace itself, or the embodiment of peace, which will end all physical conflict. We can transform ourselves or the things that surround us into beauty and healing powers or the embodiment of the waters of a river. There is no longer a separation between us and our environment, or between ourselves and other people, or other places.

Quantum physics allows us to approach the level of the Condor more easily because it has shown that matter is far from being that tangible and "solid thing" that we thought it was. The "classic" concept of matter is completely false and an illusion of the senses and mind, existing only at the level of the Puma; this is out of the question and has already been demonstrated repeatedly in laboratories and can be corroborated by any modern physicist. Matter, at its atomic level, is completely intangible, as intangible as what we call thought. And from the point of quantum physics the question then arises: "What are our thoughts composed of? Are they built or manufactured, at the subatomic level, of the same substance as "tangible" material? *And is thought and matter physically the same in the quantum field, at the subatomic level?*" That question still has no answer in the laboratories. But scientists are beginning to lean toward a definite "yes" to this question, as the "Guardians of Wisdom" have understood for thousands of years; because matter, according to Einstein's theory, is energy, and thoughts are also energy and can be transformed into things. So, if both thoughts and matter are energy, then thoughts and matter are the same. Their only difference would be in their degrees of vibration or the speed at which their internal particles move. The old thinking that "thoughts are things" is beginning to be demonstrated by quantum physics. Asking all these questions opens new ways of being in the world and brings a breath of fresh air to our existence and makes life more cheerful and optimistic. The true secret of life then, is not to be found in what is known, that which belongs to the physical level of the Serpent, but in that which is not yet known; and that is only explained at the levels of the Hummingbird and the Condor.

We really live in a world where what we see, the physical and material world, is just the tip of a huge iceberg of quantum physics that is not observable to the eyes, that deceives us all the time with visual illusions, from the level of the Serpent and the Puma. To this same huge quantum field, demonstrated today by subatomic physics, in the traditional and ancient esotericism it was called the "invisible," because there was no better name to name it. The science of subatomic reality is called "quantum physics," and is the only one that can give us answers to the reality of the "tangible" world in which we live, because it leads us to really understand this level of reality of the Condor. The older physicists, traditional and ancient, that saw bodies as solid things, belong to the levels of the Serpent and the Puma, because they were incapable of seeing otherwise.

Matter is not what we use to believe as "static and predictable." A completely false belief was that outer space was empty, and matter was solid. The truth is, that the so called "solid bodies," or "matter," that we see with our eyes and brain, are completely empty as well. The entire material world is empty. The "solid" matter we see is equally insubstantial and empty, like outer space at the atomic level. Within the atoms and molecules that make up the physical bodies, are the so called "particles" that occupy an insignificant space of the total volume of an atom or a molecule. The rest is completely "EMPTY." These particles that make up the only "solid" thing in those atoms and molecules, in turn are appearing, disappearing and disintegrating all the time. They are created and then disintegrate, and nobody knows where these particles that appear in atoms and molecules come from, nor do we know where they go when they disintegrate; only the perception at the level of the Condor can explain it.

The atom that makes up molecules and is the basis of all "solid" matter, is a small and tiny point of very dense matter at the center, and always surrounded by a murky cloud of electrons that appear and disappear constantly from physical "Existence." We don't know where they are coming from or where they are going. And equally, this core of "dense matter" appears and disappears from physical existence as fast as electrons. The most dominant theory, and close to reality, that we can deduce after knowing all this, is that this matter is completely insubstantial and rather similar to a thought, or rather a kind of concentrated bit of "information." In this way, matter could be considered as thoughts from the Supreme Creator, or of the Supreme Mind. And this solid matter in its most fundamental basis, is a kind of bit, information, or thought, that is, in turn, affected by the thought of the human being who observes or intervenes in it. This has been demonstrated with the experience of the "paradox of the lock," in physics laboratories.

When a person looks at the experiment, the "matter" behaves in a completely different way than when nobody observes it. *The observer affects the experiment with his presence, observation, and his thoughts*. Then the scientists, who have moved away from the level of the Serpent, are deducing that material things are not more "solid" than our ideas, thoughts and information. And the apparent solidity of two bodies that hit each other, is still an illusion of our senses, at the level of the Serpent or Puma.

When two "solid" bodies strike each other, the electrons that make up their atoms and molecules generate a charge that separates the electrons from the other body before there is a possibility that they would actually touch each other, and macroscopically, in the physical world, we see it as if they hit each other. Due to the advances made in the field of quantum physics, which explains the objective world that we know, what was thought to be "REAL," for example the solidity of matter, we no longer believe. And on the contrary, what we thought was "unreal," like matter is not solid, or that a body can be in two places at the same time, or that atoms appear and disappear without knowing what is happening with them, or that thought affects the behavior of an atomic particle, now we know to be REAL.

What quantum physicists have deduced by lab observations, and the "Guardians of Wisdom" discovered through their intuitions thousands of years ago, is that our perception and intention towards the world will determine its nature. The world is dreaming itself, or is programming itself, or being programmed by us, animals, animate and inanimate things. We are programming it with our mind and intentions, and thus it exists in the external as the role we play in our life, through our thoughts. Quantum physics explains how this happens. The "Guardians of Wisdom" teach us how to do it and apply it in the code "Existence" (KAWSAY). They even teach us how to intervene in matter, like how to make it rain, etc.

There are some stones at a certain temple in Cuzco, Peru, that have all their molecules arranged in one direction; this is something impossible to do with any known technology. Whoever did this, performed this action at the level of the Condor. It is not easy to modify a frightening storm or a very advanced cancer in the body of a person, but some "Guardians of Wisdom," who have been able to act from the level of the Condor, point out that, *from this timeless level, you can find that storm, or that cancer, when they are just forming, that is, before they are created, and solve them in this time. Or either find that disease or storm in the future, when it is already formed, and resolve the present in the future.* This gives rise to the concept of *circular time*, which also belongs to the tradition of the "Guardians of Wisdom" at the level of the Condor. At this level, there is no longer time, it is timeless, so we can change things before they begin to form, or in the future, when everything was solved successfully. At this level, there is only the NOW, it is not the past, nor the future. Also, at this level, we can, with intention, manipulate matter or physical phenomena, before the energy that sustains it acquires a certain physical form. This level is associated with the divine world or HANAK PACHA of the Andean people.

EXERCISE at the Level of the Condor

The Dark Violet Room

Close your eyes and think of a place of dark violet, almost black in color. Now, think that you are inside that color completely wrapped by it and have the feeling that within that color there is no distance. Everything is contained within that color-place. The most remote distance and the closest proximity exist simultaneously. There is no up or down, or inside or outside, or right or left side, or front and back. It is all contained in the very strange space you are occupying. Neither is there time. The past, present and future exists simultaneously. Maybe you feel a strange sensation because in that place there is no time or space.

When you have practiced this Exercise many times, and you have become accustomed to it, simply think of a question, or something that is happening somewhere in time, and put your mind in a state of blankness, similar to complete stillness, until you can see the answer coming to you.

CHAPTER FOURTEEN

Other Experiences at the Condor Level

An Example of a Healing done at the Level of the Condor

Imagine that a child was seized by convulsions several minutes ago. In the midst of movements and moans, a doctor arrived only to announce the words, "too late." Because the family belonged to a Methodist church, the doctor suggested that a religious minister be called. Those present were struck by horror. The mother screamed in fright and fainted. Shouts and tumults were heard everywhere. But one of those present was one of the "Guardians of Wisdom," unknown as such to the rest. He remained perfectly calm and in control. He began to sing, from the level of the "Divine Soul," but in an inaudible way; a song that his teacher had taught him. He performed the song from the higher level.

"As you are healthy in your spirit, manifest perfect health NOW in your body. See health, feel Health. Heal NOW, Now, now!"

Speaking not to the mind (Puma level); not to the human psyche (Hummingbird level); but to the "unconditioned being" in time and space, to the Divine Soul, to the immortal Spirit of the child (level of the Condor)."

He sang this song almost inaudibly, even in the midst of all the tumult that was in that place, for several minutes without ceasing. Suddenly, the convulsing limbs of the child quieted down. The little boy stopped moaning and then opened his eyes fully conscious, asking where he was?

The Andean Gratitude, "Sacred Reciprocity" AYNI is the *Essence* of the Condor Level

The Andean Code AYNI, Andean Gratitude, or "Sacred Reciprocity," is one of the most important things in the whole tradition of the "Guardians of Wisdom." The lack of Sacred Reciprocity - always taking before giving - or taking without giving back - is pettiness and is always caused by the ego. It gets stuck at the level of the Puma, preventing us from going higher and keeping us only at the level of the animals that walk on the ground. It prevents us from reaching the level of the Hummingbird, it completely prevents us from flying or "developing spiritual wings."

I point here to the description at the level of the Condor, because it is one of the essential qualities of this level that we must understand. We belong to a universal circle, where we all exist and if we lack Sacred Reciprocity, then it is essentially a lack of this understanding that prevents us from living at the Condor level.

Some common examples of this lack of Sacred Reciprocity is presented in the following words:

Whoever is negligent with their duties, who performs them unwillingly and delays them, lacks Sacred Reciprocity with others. The businessman who employs methods lacking in equity, who renders bad services or who charges more than just prices, is equally guilty of the lack of Sacred Reciprocity (Ayni). He who takes undue advantage from other people is also guilty.

Everyone in the above examples are sowing a deficient Sacred Reciprocity for the future; while the victims of these damages, caused by having taken from them an involuntary Sacred Reciprocity, are accumulating, without knowing it, in an "invisible savings account," funds, which will be delivered to them when they most need them, and with an additional interest for this same universal principle. In other traditions of "wisdom" it was also called "the principle or law of compensation."

CHAPTER FIFTEEN

The Levels of Perception in Everyday Life

Useless Solutions in the Lower Levels

Even though we can interact discerning and solving things in the four levels of perception and reality, normally, in humanity, we do it from the level of the Serpent or of the Puma. That is, the animals that move only at ground level, the lowest. Because they are the levels to which we are accustomed as a collective. They are the two lowest and "tangible" levels of reality.

From higher levels, the level of the Hummingbird and Condor, we are able to fly and see things "from above" and take Ayni as the foundation or sustenance of life. Most people usually have not received any practical instructions on this concept of life. Maybe there are many that have not even heard of them. When we get stuck at a level of low perception, at the Serpent or the Puma level, we spend a lot of time struggling with our problems. We may find many difficulties facing us and our life becomes very inefficient.

For example, if a man has an emotional conflict with his wife, he will usually try to solve the crisis by buying her some object, acting at the Serpent or material level, which makes her smile again. When someone gets depressed, they go to the shopping center and fill up with things they do not need, or they turn to food, alcohol, sex, or drugs; all of these are on the material level of the Serpent. To quench their pain, sometimes they look for some kind of distraction or fun, parties, or loud music; or they resort to risk, or danger, which gives an adrenaline high, which is the emotional level of the Puma. They take some drug recommended by the psychiatrist to simply drown their emotional pain, a solution also at the level of the Serpent. However, as we have already pointed out, these solutions at the lower levels, attached to the Earth, the Serpent or the Puma, never really work or at least not in a definitive way. Rather, they can generate addictions and greater problems.

So, at the level that we are at as a human species, we only perceive our problems, and we seek solutions to them normally from the physical reality, or at least from the level of the mind and emotions, and always in the lower levels which are attached to the Earth and the physical self. And that is why we usually fail miserably, feel powerless or weak and a victim.

But just as it is convenient to seek to understand and solve our problems more wisely from the highest level, at the Hummingbird and Condor levels, we can equally solve our problems on all levels simultaneously. The important thing, or the key, is to *never neglect the level at which the situation or problem was created*.

For example, if someone is sick, she can act on the four levels of perception and action simultaneously. At the level of the Serpent, it is treated with proper diet, minerals, antioxidants, vitamins, medicinal herbs, thermal baths, compresses, massages, Exercises, colon therapy, cold or heat therapies, electricity or magnetism and medications. At the level of the Puma, it can be treated with analysis, psychology or mental suggestions. At the Hummingbird level, it can be treated with meditation, ritual acts, crepuscular states, evolutionary therapy, hypnotherapy, healing visualizations and psycho-magical acts or spiritual practices. And at the Condor level, you can treat the problem with your conscience and wisdom of the Divine Spirit or with magical acts. Also, do not seek to develop the powers of the Hummingbird or the Condor from the levels of the ego or the Puma, or to put them at the feet of the ego, because then the results you get will not be satisfactory. They will not have enough sustenance of Ayni and all the good obtained will be corrupt or deviated and will bring misfortune to others and finally, even more, to oneself.

Trying to Seek the Divine from a Lower Level

Many people try to apply religious dogmas that correspond only to the level of the Puma, to obtain the development of the Soul and the Spirit; that is, to embrace dogmas that are at the levels of the Hummingbird or the Condor while still at the level of the Puma. This simply is not possible. Because when we try to solve a problem at a higher level from a lower level it simply does not work. It is like trying to tie a cloud with a string, or to solve a psychosomatic illness, generated by the mind and emotions, with drugs, surgery or electroshock.

The Realization of the Poet Rumi

Rumi, the great Sufi mystic and poet, once told the story of how
he knocked on the door of his beloved God:

"Who is there?" Was the answer.
"It's me, your lover, Rumi," he said.

From inside the voice came out,
"Go away, there's no
place or space for the two of us here."
Rumi left, completely discouraged.
He meditated and prayed, and then
he returned to his beloved's house
once again and knocked on the door.
"Who is it?" The beloved asked.
"I am You."
With a great welcome, the door opened
wide.

While Rumi searched for God with his ego, holding on with his dogmas and with a sense of separation of time and space and his material personality, he could not get in. Only when he climbed to the level of the Condor and turned away from the ideas of separation and duality, did he achieve it fully.

The History of Brother Daniel

Every morning at 4 a.m., Brother Daniel was the first to get up in the monastery. He got up early of his own accord, and he was proud to do so. While his teacher and all his brothers slept peacefully, Brother Daniel actively exerted great effort in his practices of prayer, study and meditation. Illumination was his goal.

Every day, Brother Daniel prayed more and more intensely for illumination. He worked very hard to improve his physical posture in meditation, and, above all, he worked to memorize all the ancient spiritual texts. Rarely, did Brother Daniel rest, eat or sleep, because he wanted to reach illumination and he wanted to get there quickly. Brother Daniel liked to meditate and pray, but above all, he immersed himself in the scriptures. He liked to be quiet and immobile, but rarely had time, because he discovered that there was always much to do. He liked silence, but he would prefer to hear his teacher talk about silence. Brother Daniel's teacher was a kind and peaceful man who was always smiling, encouraging Brother Daniel to slow down, enjoy the sun and watch the grass grow. But Brother Daniel was too interested in chasing an ideal and in too much of a hurry to obtain illumination to pay attention to his teacher's advice. "Why do you hurry, accelerate and rush so much?" Asked his teacher one day. "I am looking for illumination," replied Brother Daniel. His teacher smiled. "When will you get there?" "Oh, one more prayer perhaps, or in my next meditation, or in an act of service perhaps," replied Brother Daniel. "Why are you so sure that illumination is running ahead of you?" asked his teacher.

"Maybe if you stopped for a moment, you would find that illumination is already here right now with you, chasing after you, trying to catch up to you, but you are so busy moving forward that you do not give it time to reach you!"

As long as Brother Daniel searched from his ego, he could not get what he found on the level of the Condor.

CHAPTER SIXTEEN

The Problem of Unhappiness

The Futility of Seeking Happiness in the Lower Levels of the Serpent and the Puma

People usually seek the solution to happiness from a wrong level of reality, from the lower level, and again they fail. They look for it from the level of the Serpent, physical conditions, or from the mind and emotions, the level of the Puma, building around it a large number of mistaken mental and emotional beliefs and associations, "true fantasies." This is because the two lower levels of reality are like the Puma or the Serpent that know no more than the level of the ground, which is very strongly conditioned to time and space. Happiness does not exist there. For these reasons it is completely impossible to solve the problem of human unhappiness from the level of the Serpent, the material, or from the level of the Puma, the mind and emotions. Authentic happiness is only found or resolved from the level of the Condor, the spiritual level. It is on this level, that it appears spontaneously without any additional effort on the part of anyone.

We can attend many seminars on happiness but if we search from the lower reality levels, we will not advance an inch towards it. When searching from the material or from the mind and emotions, which corresponds to the levels of the Serpent and the Puma, we usually put requirements and conditions, or physical or mental demands and solutions, on what we call "happiness." This generates by itself frustration, and the exact opposite to what we are looking for, in such a way that a constant unhappiness is generated. This is because we are putting material, mental and emotional conditions on that goal, seeking to resolve it at those levels, where it is not possible for happiness to exist.

Some of the conditions or material solutions, at the level of the Serpent, that we usually put on happiness are:

"I will get happiness when I meet a suitable partner, or have the right job, or the right profession, or reach certain achievements related to my body or money. Or, when I live in a certain place, city, country, area, or house, or have more "free time."

All these chimerical solutions to achieve happiness are placed from the level of the

Serpent, the physical and material. Time set as a condition for happiness also constitutes a completely physical measurement, such as goods, work, place, and conditions. As proof that these conditions or solutions to find happiness from matter, at the level of the Serpent, are only illusions, let us remember once again that for society in general, the last decades were the decades of acquiring the "most" in the material world. People tried to buy happiness by acquiring more "things" and a "dream" of an ideal material life. Contradictory to what was expected, society became more depressed, more violent, more suicidal and more stressed than ever. Society moved in the opposite direction by doing this. This shows that seeking to resolve happiness from the lower level is never a solution.

If someone wants to reach it, then he must do as those who have achieved it; this is, look for happiness only from the upper level of the Condor, the level of our "unconditioned being" or timelessness. Our unconditioned being, or Divine Soul, does not demand any material condition, nor time, nor space, to be eternally happy. Living life at the level of the Puma, we put all kinds of conditions of time and space to something that is not physical like happiness. So, if we really want happiness, it is absurd to assign material conditions and say, "when I live in that place" (space condition), or "when I have made enough effort," and I have "earned it" (time condition), then I will be happy. Because it is as impractical as asking our partner to give us "60 decibels of red flowers" on Valentine's Day. Could your partner meet your conditions? They certainly could not do it, because it's impossible. A material thing like flowers cannot be measured in terms of decibels or sound.

Negative Self-Talk

Other causes of unhappiness are because we are mentally, and subconsciously, trapped in a network at the Puma level, with thoughts and emotions linked to:

> "low self-esteem,"
> "not being good enough,"
> "having been wrong,"
> "being guilty of something in the past,"
> "being bad,"
> or "not accepting ourselves."

We can know if we have this problem by doing the test of staying alone with ourselves a whole day or a full weekend. Another experiment is to find if it is difficult or uncomfortable to remain silent when being next to a person who is not close to us. If we have this problem, we have a lack of acceptance at the Puma level. All those false conditions lead us to think and feel that:

"we do not deserve happiness,"
"we are not worthy of it,"
"it is not easy to obtain it,"
"it is only achieved with a lot of effort after a long time,"
"only when we have paid the price," or
"worked enough for it" or anything else.

In this mental and emotional level of the puma, we have subconsciously conditioned ourselves that it is really "not good or practical to be happy" or we learned to be afraid of happiness because "we will feel bad to see that there are so many people who are not happy." More common negative thoughts are:

"we will awaken the envy of others,"
"they will hate us and persecute us for being happy,"
"we will feel guilty for that," or
"how can we have the gall to be happy if others are not?"

Equally, the mere fact of thinking that "we need happiness," or "we pray for it," is also subconsciously conditioning the mind to a thought of unhappiness, because the mind creates our reality. Through all these thoughts, associations and conditioning, we have programmed ourselves to be in a constant state of unhappiness. It will be impossible to overcome, no matter how many courses or seminars on happiness we attend. Because the unhappiness we are trying to solve at the level of the Serpent or Puma is a true condition or mental illness that cannot be healed with seminars or courses. It requires a "subconscious reconditioning," as all the limiting constraints of the mind must experience.

This explains why millions of people living in prosperity and physical health and having everything that could be designated as "ideal material life," continue to feel unhappy and miserable. They are trying to obtain in the material level something that is timeless and without space, immaterial, like happiness. The ego, besides erring in its search, generally creates a platform of reality that is completely contradictory or hindering at the level of the Condor. And so, it develops concepts such as "separability," "individual good," a "competition" that gives rise to selfishness, or a "personal, group or racial superiority" from which springs pride. *This false pride is the worst of all human evils, because it gives rise to all the others.*

At the level of the Condor there is the concept of "unity" in all things and the "welfare of others," through the Andean Code of Sacred Reciprocity, or AYNI, in all things, or the Christian's Golden Rule. "Always do to others what you want them to do to you," this dissolves selfishness. It conceptualizes the idea that the Divine is in everyone, without distinction, and it also has the power to destroy pride and vanity. For this reason, before being initiated in the Temple of the Condor, the highest of all levels, the aspirant to the level of the "guardian of the wisdom" in the Andes, had to pass through the initiations or "purifications" of the Temple of the Puma. In the Temple of the Puma, if he wanted to get to fly once again in the incredible heights of the Condor, he had to dissolve the moorings of the illusory matrix of his ego.

CHAPTER SEVENTEEN

Reinforcing the Ideas of the Mistakes Committed at the Different Levels of Reality

Lower Levels Can Drag the Activity of Higher Levels Down

Occasionally we can perceive things from the level of the Hummingbird or the Condor, but then the physical perception of the level of the Serpent can drag us backwards, make us retreat, like when we believe that we do not have enough time or money. Or, we go to the level of the Puma and we doubt our capabilities. Or, we run the risk of putting the great powers of the Hummingbird and the Condor at the feet of the ego on the level of the Puma, bringing misery and dissatisfaction on all sides. At the level of the Condor, our power to change reality is at its zenith. However, the level of the Puma can make us descend, pointing out that we need courage and practice to reach this higher level of perception and stay there.

Looking for Solutions to Our Problems From the Highest Levels-
These are the Most Efficient Solutions

The "Guardians of Wisdom" quickly learn to diagnose and cure diseases and negative conditions which include life problems such as bad luck, deficient affective relationships, and many more from the level of the Hummingbird. This is one of the best levels to work in, especially if the cause of such diseases is at the level of the human soul, or psyche, which manifests itself below into the physical body. They do not work physically with the body, level of the Serpent, or psychologically with the mind, level of the Puma, when the disease was created at the level of the human soul or psyche level of the Hummingbird. We can affirm as a universal law that:

Every problem we face must be resolved at the level at which it was created. Generally, to a level higher than that in which it
manifested. Because if we do it only at the level that they manifested, there will only be a temporary solution or none at all. But from the level of the Condor EVERYTHING is healed.

If the disease or problem, for example, is an allergy, or economic problems, and it was created at the Puma level, by trapped emotions, guilt or fear, it should be resolved at the level of the Hummingbird, since the problem originated at the level of the Puma. The "Guardians of Wisdom" work at the Hummingbird level with rituals, logical acts or "psycho-magic," where personal altars, feathers, herbs, drums, dances, movements, words, and fire are present. They also use other symbolic or metaphorical tools of the Hummingbird level that allow them to heal at the level of the human soul or psyche. These methods can complement the procedures at the same physical level with massages, baths of florid water, sun baths and other movements. But the most experienced do not need to use any of this because they work from the level of the Condor, where objects, rituals, illogical acts or thoughts and visual images, are not necessary. They can heal with a prayer or an invocation to a Divine Being of power, like Pachamama, who is the Mother of all life and existence (Mother of Nature), and who is inseparable from the Godhead, or to the sacred beings of the mountains who are called, "**Apus.**" The most advanced among the Guardians can, with only their mere presence, apply with "certainty and intention," the healing process or a solution to a problem.

We see this also in the Gospels of Jesus, who was a great adherent to the practice of Sacred Reciprocity. In some cures, Jesus acted at the level of the Hummingbird of the human soul, or psyche, with metaphors or illogical "rituals" such as mixing his saliva with Earth and putting this mud over the eyes of a blind man. But then he also acted at the level of the Condor, healing a sick person with only his spoken voice. And finally, he did nothing, not making any effort, just with his very presence. A woman, who suffered from constant uterine bleeding, that did not yield to any treatment, was healed without his intervening when she touched the robe of Jesus.

If we are working on ourselves at the level of the Hummingbird, we can solve a melancholy or depressive mood by singing happy songs, as the philosopher Marcelo Ficino suggested during the Renaissance and Dr. Gerard Encausse during the Belle Epoque in Paris. We can also improve our situation by dressing in clothes of white color, bright colors, or reciting prayers, hoping that uttering magic words will lead us to truly feel good. At the top level of the Condor, we will not need any of these things, because we can pass from the level of the Hummingbird, to those practices belonging to the level of the Condor, and experience the "unconditional and timeless being" that we are; then, our mood will change in a very different way at this higher level. From the level of the Condor you can cure all the lower levels, all situations, and not have to use the tools of the other levels, because it will be enough. So, it is said that Simon the Magician, so respected among the Romans, who operated only from the level of the Hummingbird, with rituals, magical and illogical acts, asked Peter to teach him, in exchange for a lot of money, how to operate at the superior level of the Condor, that he did not understand. Because he realized that it was a very "superior magic" to which Peter knew, and which was much more powerful, with far reaching results, and with less effort.

The Hummingbird with all its virtues and powers, however desirable, cannot be compared with the high level of the Condor and the heights in which it lives. There are different levels among the "Guardians of Wisdom" of the Andes. There are the Paqos and the Teqse Paqos. The **Paqos** are considered as teachers of the third level of consciousness, and the **Teqse Paqos** who teach from the fourth level of consciousness upwards. The first, among which most of the Queros are found, solve their problems and practice medicine from the Hummingbird's reality. But the Teqse Paqos are very rare and seek to solve their own problems and other´s from the level of the Condor.

Understand and Solve Your Problems from the Highest Levels...

But Lower Levels Should Not Be Discarded

When your perception goes to a higher level, like the Hummingbird and the Condor, you can transform the many problems you may have in the physical and emotional world. For this reason, of the four symbolic animals of reality levels, only two fly: the Hummingbird and the Condor. The Serpent and the Puma move at ground level, which is why they represent their vision and ability, in a much smaller capacity.

As you rise above the level of perception of those problems and perceive it with the eye of the "ñawi" of higher perception, you may understand that what appears to be a problem at the lower level, is really an opportunity. The Chinese of antiquity who developed their language millennia ago show that they had highly developed ñawis of higher perception at the Hummingbird and Condor levels, because the word crisis in Chinese "Wei Ji" is formed by those two characters. The first is Wei, which means danger and the second is Ji, which means opportunity.

For example, losing a job, or ending a loving relationship with someone which is at the Puma level, looks like an enormous tragedy, but it can be a tremendous opportunity to renew ourselves from the perspective of the Hummingbird and the Condor that has vision from above. The same with a disease which gives you the opportunity to experience a profound transformation and know yourself better. From the level of the Hummingbird, we always observe the silver lining in a dark cloud. While from the Puma level we usually only observe the dark mass of that cloud.

One of my teachers, who had always been very delicate in health, constantly told me that the disease had been his best friend. He always said that, thanks to his illness and ailments, he was still alive, and he lived to an old age. In his youth he had given himself up to certain excesses, in food and fun. When he got sick, he could not continue his dissipated lifestyle. It also made him re-think about the goal of life, which later led him to contact "Guardians of Wisdom."

Going to a higher level of perception allows us to recognize that by protecting a species from extinction, we not only do so with that species, but with all of nature. This is something global, and at the same time, we deliver the message of responsibility and care to humanity. From the level of the Hummingbird and the Condor, we can understand the hidden connection in all things in nature and perceive the synchronicities that are everywhere. At these levels we learn that *there are no coincidences* and that everything has a purpose and a meaning.

The four centers of inferior perception, however, are also useful at certain times. When you face danger in an isolated place, you can access the level of the Serpent, put aside your fear and use the cold and emotionless resources of the reptilian brain to control the pain of your broken leg. The Serpent, which is cold and indifferent, allows you to instinctively take care of your wound until you can get back on the road and find someone to help you. The perception of the Serpent is equally useful in an emergency that involves several people, like responding to a fire, or an earthquake. The cold blood of the Serpent can be extremely useful and valuable here. This lower level can prevent us from falling into possible fantasies, false philosophies or utopias at the level of the Hummingbird. Avoiding this path, we can separate a life from fantasy, as mentioned in another section of this book. Also, the Serpent makes us develop a sense of "security," and to work and save, so that there are no shortcomings in our lives. In that sense, it is quite practical because we need to pay the bills, clean up, and take the children to school, without looking for any other meaning to these acts. At this level, before any crisis arises, we seek to have money in the bank, or in safe deposit box, or in gold coins. The Serpent seeks security without losing energy, thinking about the issues, analyzing or anguishing for their cause, which corresponds to the Puma. A person who refuses to function at this level, believes that the material Serpent can be impractical in their life.

At the Puma level you can experience many feelings including fear and vulnerability. But when you climb to the level of the Hummingbird, you begin to have a higher vision. You become aware of the connection between your broken leg, in that isolated place, and perhaps of too many responsibilities. You understand that in order to be able to heal permanently, and not to have accidents of this kind again, you're going to have to stop wanting to have control of all the details in life, and trust more in the laws of the Universe. If you only heal the leg you will only have a temporary relief from just that accident, you will not have healed from the level at which this situation was created, the level of the human soul or psyche. The next time you might break the other leg, or you will have another type of accident, until you cure the cause in that level of the mind and emotions. Because…

Every problem we face must be resolved at the level at which it was created; generally, at a level higher than that in which it manifests.

If we do it only at the level that the problem manifests, there will only be a temporary solution, or none at all.

But from the level of the Condor EVERYTHING is healed.

From the perspective of the Condor, you will be able to mentally project yourself, leaving the current time and space, and then going into the future to find a better outcome than dying alone in that isolated region. It is here that you will be able to choose a better destination, one where a ranger comes to help you. At the level of the Condor, you can also recognize that healing does not only involve the body, but also the Divine Soul, or Immortal Spirit, the "unconditioned being," that longs to meet with the experiences that he came to get on Earth; including the reason for having injured the body at that moment and in that isolated place.

But if you have entered the path of the "guardians of knowledge," you must be faithful to it and must not abandon it as soon as you begin to feel physically and emotionally, at the levels of the Serpent and the Puma, with the tools you learn. Observing things from the level of the Hummingbird allows you to understand that feeling good is convenient, but that evolving to the level of the Condor, unfolding all your potential as a human and a divine being, is much more important. It is the destiny of every human being who treads on Earth. And by observing with the eyes of the Condor, it is understood that by reaching its power, we can begin to *dream our world* and translate it into concrete reality. *Our own personal development is related to the evolution and healing of the entire planet. We are all linked together by invisible ties, and we all have a common destiny and that is to come together at the highest level.*

Usually, all programs of personal development, coaching, self-help and the like, aim only to satisfy the ego and to have great success and excellence at the levels of the Serpent and the Puma. They aim to fully satisfy those levels only, and not beyond. They never lead us to a real state of happiness, because happiness is at the level of the Condor. I myself have been for many years a hypnotherapist and an international coach, and I have found that only the training of the "Guardians of Wisdom" of the Andes, points to the highest qualities of our being, the levels of the Hummingbird and the Condor.

Another advantage of being able to move through the different levels of perception and work in them, is the fact that if you are destined to experience a deadly hereditary disease, you do not have to live it on the physical level, where you would end up developing it. At the level of the Hummingbird, you can avoid it by learning the lessons it has come to teach you, through what I call "evolutionary therapy." In the Condor you can clean the codes in your "luminous energy sphere," that contain the ill conditions, such as a genetic disease, and visualize a different past or future for yourself. You can also, by moving through the different levels of reality, make your ideas descend from the levels of the Condor or Hummingbird, through the symbolization and materialization with the "Existence" and "Wisdom" Codes and make it come true in your life.

Although naturally we feel more attracted to a certain level of reality and their perceptions, and work in it with perseverance, we must learn to be the master of all four levels. Some Exercises in this book will help you develop your ability to work your way through them and move freely in the four levels of reality, with all their perceptions and powers. By continually living and working with all four levels, which we are naturally designed as human beings to do since the beginning of time, we become conscious of the powers and talents given to us by the Creator. We came into the world with the four perception centers, that are called ñawis, to assist us with our journey into eternity. There are no human beings who lacks them. We all live simultaneously in the four realities.

Four Levels of Reality

To summarize these teachings, there are four types of perceptions of them through which the "Guardians of Wisdom of the Andes" come into contact with the four levels of reality. These levels correspond to the four dimensions of the general Universe of vibration and light.

1) The material world, represented in a human being by our physical body, symbolized by the Serpent;
2) the realm of concrete mind, represented in a human being by his thoughts, the ideas and emotions associated with them at the level of the Puma;
3) the realm of the semi-Divine, represented in a human being by our psyche or human soul, in the Hummingbird kingdom of the mythical world;
4) and finally, the non-physical Divine world represented in a human being by the Immortal Spirit, his Divine Soul, "unconditioned being" or primordial energy, represented by the Condor.

CHAPTER EIGHTEEN

Vehicles in a Human Being Belonging to the Four Levels of Reality

The Human Being is a Small Universe

The four levels of reality, the different vehicles of manifestation in the human being, establish four centers of perception, associated, as I have pointed out, with a physical center in the brain. The vehicles in the human being transport and individualize the universal activity of each world, or reality, in a human being, thus transforming it into a replica of the Universe itself. This is known as the small universe or "microcosm."

The 4 Human Vehicles

The ordering of these 4 human vehicles, from the densest to the subtlest and from the hierarchically inferior to the hierarchically superior, are organized in the following way:

1. First, the physical body as the grossest form, is the innermost part and of the lowest hierarchy in this scale of vehicles. The physical body is

like a mooring anchor for the other subtler and hierarchically superior vehicles. Intimately linked to it, but in a slightly higher hierarchical order, is the electro-vital or etheric vehicle, also called the "vehicle of the formative forces," which surrounds the physical body, following its contour. It is an autonomous entity; whose function is to preserve the physical body from disintegration. It is composed of electromagnetism, electric and magnetic force (yin yang), which has also been called "vitality or life," Chi, Qi, and Prana in oriental cultures.

"These two lower vehicles correspond to the level of the Serpent. The first, completely made of matter, linked to the physical level, and in direct relation to the world of matter, that feeds it. The second, etheric-vital or electromagnetic body, feeds from the vital electric and magnetic world, Chi, Qi, Prana."

2. Less dense than the previous vehicles, but directly influencing them to be hierarchically in a higher position, is a body that some people call the sidereal, or astral, and whose purpose is to animate the physical body and serve as a "matrix" of

connection for the inferior mind with the higher levels of consciousness. It is used to connect the sensations between the physical and the mental and to be able to communicate activity of that higher level to the physical body and vice versa. Its hierarchy is superior to the previous one and less dense. It is also the mental-emotional body that some have called the "animal soul." These two make up the level of the Puma (mental-emotional).

3. Hierarchically superior to the previous ones, and less dense, is the human soul, or the psychic vehicle, or the "Psyche" level; that is a vehicle of connection between the Divine Soul, or Immortal Spirit, and the lower level of the mental-emotional body and this corresponds to the level of the Hummingbird. This vehicle of the human soul, or psyche, is immersed and feeds on the "symbolic world," and the electro-vital body of prana, or chi, much like the body feeds on physical food.

4. And finally, at the highest and subtler of all, is the Divine Soul or Immortal Spirit, the "unconditioned being" that corresponds to the level of the Condor. It is the real being, the true SELF. It is not affected by time or space. It is immersed and involved in the essential world; that is, in its own immortal or Divine reality. It feeds directly from the higher Divine energies, and from Divine thoughts directly, and lives under the higher universal principles such as Sacred Reciprocity or AYNI.

The "Luminous Energy Sphere"

The Human Being as a Passenger, Coachman, Horse and Carriage

George Ivanovich Gurdjieff and Dr. Gerard Encausse made a representation of the human being divided into 4 parts, but they represented it under the metaphor of a passenger, a coachman, a horse and a carriage. Giving them the same attributes that we have seen here in this book at the four levels of the "Guardians of Wisdom."

1)Passenger (level of the Condor),

2) a coachman (level of the Hummingbird),

3) a horse (level of the Puma) and

4) carriage (level of the Serpent, or physical body).

The set of all these parts of the vehicles, or levels of universal expression in a human being, which envelop the physical body, is the central anchor, which finally receives all these influences as an obedient receiver, and a corporal manifestation of the previous ones, or a passive and receptive vessel of everything above. They wrap the physical body as a cloud of subtle energies, called the Human Aura, and in the Quechua language "Poqpo," "bubble," or "sphere of luminous energy."

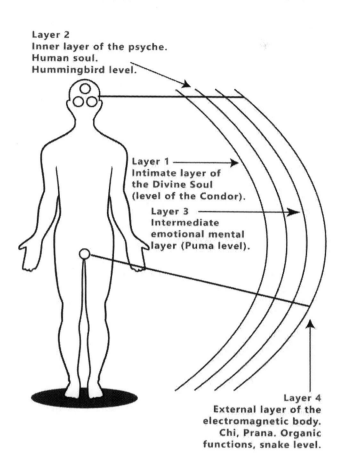

Layer 2
Inner layer of the psyche.
Human soul.
Hummingbird level.

Layer 1
Intimate layer of
the Divine Soul
(level of the Condor).

Layer 3
Intermediate
emotional mental
layer (Puma level).

Layer 4
External layer of the
electromagnetic body.
Chi, Prana. Organic
functions, snake level.

As noted, the physical body is then wrapped in a true cloud of energies composed of four layers. They are inlaid, assembled, or embedded within each other, as do the Russian Babushka dolls inside each other. It is all completely mixed in this "sphere of luminous energy," or POQPO.

Four Levels of the Luminous Energy Sphere

These four layers, in the "sphere of luminous energy," are not really separated from each other, in the same way that the colors of the rainbow are not separated from each other, but rather they are diluted and interpenetrate in each other. Simply put, the denser energies manifest themselves more on the surface by decantation, or separation, as the oil that is denser is naturally separated from the water when we mix it. The oil separates naturally to form the outer surface because of its greater density.

By observing this "sphere of luminous energy," we thus detect 4 layers or "radiations," that extend from the material body. These layers, from the inside out, by "decantation," correspond to the following levels:

1. The most intimate or internal to the level of the Spirit. Also known as Divine Soul (the level of the Condor).

2. Internal to the level of the higher mind or psyche. Also known as human soul (the level of the Hummingbird).
3. The middle one, at the emotional mind level, also called "animal soul" (the level of the Puma).

4. The most external to the physical corresponds to the electro vital or etheric body, which prevents the disintegration of the same (the level of the Serpent).

Luminous Energy Sphere from Outside Inward

Each layer mixed with the others but separated from the next by "density and decantation," stores a different type of energy. As water and oil don't mix completely, they are decanting towards the outside according to their greater density. We will *review the different layers from the* **outside inwards**.

4. The outermost (**layer 4/ Serpent**) is the densest and accumulates the energy provided

by electromagnetism, prana, Chi, Qi, Kausay, which nourishes the physical body with life and prevents its disintegration and fulfills organic functions. The codes or records of a physical trauma or disease are stored in the outer, dense layer, or layer 4 (Serpent) of our "sphere of luminous energy," and there it establishes the CAUSES of our illnesses or accidents.

3. The next, inner is (**layer 3/ Puma**) less dense than the previous one, stores the energies that support the mental and emotional resistance. Codes of emotional records, or imprints, are stored in the next layer, layer 3 (Puma,) and there it establishes the CAUSES or ORIGINS of certain emotional dysfunctions. This is due to the emotional interpretations and distorted meanings that we make of the world and our life. But these emotional dysfunctions bring an even greater problem than the physical one, and can also, if not treated in time, descend through the vehicle or "matrix" of connections between mind and body, called the astral body, and finally manifest an illness or accident in the physical body.

2. Beneath it, even less dense is (**layer 2/ Hummingbird**) the psychic energy of the human soul, psyche or higher mind. Codes or records of the human soul, higher mind, or psyche (layer 2) are stored in the next layer

which is the Hummingbird level, and there they establish the CAUSE or ORIGIN of certain mental anomalies. These are mental creations of the past, which are distorted imaginations. But these anomalies, because they are higher than the emotional mental level, can also in time by descending through the vehicle or "matrix" of connections between human soul and mind-emotion, manifest at the level of emotional dysfunctions, whose cause is of a psychic type. If not resolved in good time, they will also generate, or manifest, an illness or accident, on the physical level, even though its original cause is at the level of the higher mind, human soul or psyche - the Hummingbird.

1. The subtlest of all (**layer 1/ Condor**) the most intimate layer, corresponds to the radiations coming from the Immortal Spirit, the "unconditioned being," or "Divine Soul." Codes or records of past lives, which contain our actions in the distant past, good or bad, and the amount of AYNI, or lack of it, with which we have lived in the past, is recorded here on the Condor level. And here, is established the CAUSE or ORIGIN of certain anomalies by "indebtedness with the Divine level" that can appear in all the lower levels; including the psychic-mental, emotional or physical levels of our life. These causes can only be dissolved with SACRED RECIPROCITY, kindness and

sincere prayer; they depend on divine causes directly related to God, or the Source of Everything.

The sphere of luminous energy thus contains in each of its layers, separated by density, registered in its energy codes, all the personal and ancestral memories of good and bad experiences of the past and previous lives. These records, codes or imprints are stored in codes of different colors and intensities. Records, codes or imprints are like computer programs and when they are activated, they determine dysfunctional behaviors, mentally, emotionally and behaviorally, but they can also produce accidents and illnesses. According to the "Guardians of Wisdom," our personal history is repeated in cycles.

CHAPTER NINETEEN

Shape of the "Luminous Energy Sphere"
Understanding Our Aura of Light and Energy

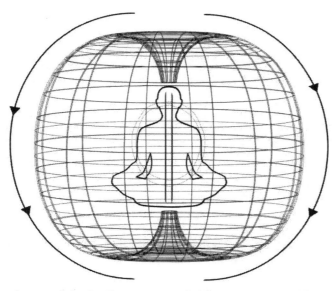

Image of the luminous energy field currents created by
the Kausay in a human being.
The energies of Kausay enter below and go out above
to enter below again creating a kind of toroid field in
every human being.

The shape of our "luminous energy sphere"
is what in geometry is called "torus;" it's similar

to a "doughnut," with a very narrow central hole in the center.

The energies of this "sphere of Luminous energy," (Kausay) rise up from the legs through our physical body to the top of the head. They expand through our open arms and then down the outside of the body to go back up the legs. This is done in the 360 degrees around the physical body, in all directions of space, forming a kind of "doughnut" or geometric torus. This is the physical form of our "Luminous energy sphere."

Modern Life and the Luminous Energy Sphere

When we live in a very populated city, this "donut" usually collapses, tightens and narrows enormously, like a very tight chrysalis around the physical body. But when we are in nature, in the open air, we return to our natural state, and this "Luminous energy field" widens again and regains its normal size.

The "Luminous energy sphere" becomes poisonous or toxic when we make negative interpretations of reality, or when we make our mind toxic with distorted thoughts and beliefs about life. For this reason, we have methods to de-tox or remove negative emotions that we are not able to properly process or clean normally. These negative thoughts and images begin to form in our luminous sphere at the different levels or layers (psychic, mental, emotional), as psychic mud, or stagnant energies. They begin to weaken us, slow down, and even stop the flow of energies in our "luminous energy sphere." They also can reverse their currents and alter the entire circulation of these fluid energies. Stagnant energies, if not dealt with, will give rise to different alterations and damages, manifesting finally at the physical level as diseases. If we do not give attention to these "energy stagnations," (Hucha in Quechua tongue) our physical body will not increase very much its vitality and prolong its life. Since at the purely physical level, the level of the Serpent, our cells have an enormous power of regeneration; we naturally and spontaneously regenerate. Through this natural regenerative capacity, a new copy of our bodies is regenerated every eight months when the old cells die and are replaced by new and younger ones. Weakness, diseases and premature aging are produced by alterations and intoxication carried out by us in our thoughts, emotions, and acts, in our sphere of luminous energy.

Codes or Records in the "Luminous Energy Sphere"

A *record, or code, is an impact that occurs in one of the levels of reality and that will generate an organization of information in the "luminous energy sphere" that will shape our mental, emotional and physical world.* The information contained in a code of the "luminous energy sphere" shapes the sphere that, in turn, organizes the physical body. We can thus see that these different levels of perceptions of reality are equally organized in layers in the sphere, embedded within each other. They inform the other levels from within. The Immortal Spirit, or Divine Soul, informs or governs the human soul (higher mind, psyche or Hummingbird level), which informs and governs the emotional mind (Puma level) and this eventually informs and finally governs, the physical body (level of the Serpent).

This "luminous energy sphere," Kausay, in its different levels, or layers, is organizing the lower levels, until reaching the physical body, which is the densest level, in the same way that the energy fields of a magnet orders the iron scrapings that have been deposited on a sheet of paper. The "Guardians of Wisdom," in this way, discovered that to really help to heal a human being, one must be familiar with, and work on, the four levels of reality, independently or simultaneously in them. The aim of this book has been to explain this process.

In this "luminous energy sphere" is the mold, plan or blueprint of the way in which we should live, on how we age and how we might die. When there is no disease code in the "luminous energy sphere," the person will recover from any disease at a tremendous speed. In the same way, the codes or imprints of diseases can depress the immune system by itself and it may take a lot longer to recover health. If that code is not deleted, this disease, situation, or problem can be repeated in cycles.

The "Guardians of Wisdom" learned to heal diseases and create extraordinary health states, to maintain physical youth, as well as to shape and transform their individual destinies by improving this "luminous energy sphere." This "luminous energy sphere," at its densest levels, finally instructs the DNA and body chemistry of the body. If we can erase the negative trace that caused the onslaught of the immune system, we can eradicate the disease at a tremendous speed. This knowledge allows us to access this "luminous energy sphere" directly, or indirectly, through the practices contained in this book, and to create a new sphere that in the densest levels physically forms a new body that ages, regenerates, and dies in a different way.

Many forms of healing used by the "Guardians of Wisdom" always intervened directly or indirectly with this "luminous energy sphere." As shown in this book, it is necessary to understand that the causes of our problems have origins, manifestations in each of the different levels of reality, as they are manifested in the records within the "luminous energy sphere." If it is programmed for disease, and we only intervene at the physical level, as do those who only perceive the physical reality at the level of the Serpent, through surgeries or medications - there may be a re-occurring manifestation of the problem. It is not going to heal, or is going to re-appear, or manifest itself in another way, perhaps even worse. Without improving, positively modifying, reprogramming or healing this "luminous energy sphere," we are trapped in the codes of past suffering and even genetic inheritance, at the physical level of the Serpent; that is, we age and die in the same way as our parents and grandparents have done, reliving their physical illnesses and emotional disorders. By becoming "Guardians of Wisdom" we also reject any ideology or politics that values control and domination over nature, which justifies the exploitation of rivers and forests and does not respect the lives of other beings, because it sees them only as resources for the human consumption. Instead, we adopt a thousand-year-old wisdom and ideology, which is ancient and timeless, that most human beings have lost, which is love, cooperation and sustainability between all life forms.

Understanding the contents of this book and its corresponding practices will help you change your perceptions, dream a new world and make it come true in a way that you would not have thought possible before. Through this knowledge imparted by the "Guardians of Wisdom," humanity has the ability to evolve, not between generations, but within a single generation, which contradicts the knowledge we had so far on human evolution. It also can eradicate from our inner centers, vortices, ñawis and chakras, the seed roots of bad habits, inclinations and negative tendencies, that would generate future ills, in a cyclical way, and correct the negative programs that lead to old age, disease and death.

CHAPTER TWENTY

The Human Being as a Temple or House

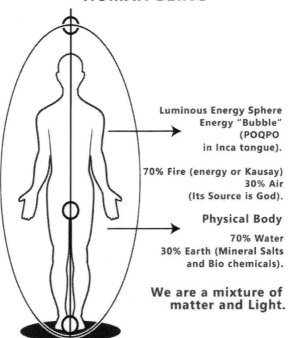

**"Wasi" (House of "Temple")
HUMAN BEING**

Luminous Energy Sphere
Energy "Bubble"
(POQPO
in Inca tongue).

70% Fire (energy or Kausay)
30% Air
(Its Source is God).

Physical Body

70% Water
30% Earth (Mineral Salts
and Bio chemicals).

**We are a mixture of
matter and Light.**

Luminous Energy Sphere

According to the Andean wisdom, we are composed simultaneously of light (energy) and matter (Earth). The light or energy of which we are composed forms around us what is called "Energy Bubble" or "Luminous Energy Sphere," or "Toroid," which surrounds our bodies in a diameter of up to 2 meters (6 feet). Don Joaquin and many other Andean masters called it -in ancient tongue- "POQPO." In it are all the codes and records that determine our life, our health, our economic well-being, our emotional relationships and our "good or bad luck." It is also responsible for our mental, emotional and physical health integrity. Through it, we learn to heal ourselves, mentally, emotionally, and physically, and to heal others, and finally, to heal the world. It is the true plane or "blueprint" that determines our life; the kind of life we have and will lead, unless we program it in another way, which can be done, and is part of training in the Andean tradition. But that is not all…

Through the sphere of light energy, or POQPO, we are connected in their different layers with all the rest of the Universe, visible and invisible, with other human beings, with the stars, with the planets, with the rocks, with the plants, with animals, and with all the energies that surround us in our environment and with the material world, electromagnetic, celestial, and finally the Divine. Even in certain ways, we are connected with things that are very far from us; such as places, temples, people and beings. In this sphere of luminous energy, one of its outer layers is formed of a substance or energy called "Existence," (Kausay) that gives existence to all things and all beings in the Universe. This "Existence" can be composed of very fine and fluid energy or heavy or stagnant energy. Only human beings can have heavy or stagnant energy in their spheres of luminous energy; the animals, the stars, the rocks, the trees, only have fluid energy.

The energy of this sphere, in a healthy, optimistic and cheerful person, is always fluid; but if it is full of sadness, anger, bitterness or any of the harmful emotions, this energy stagnates. When it remains a long time stagnant, it finally forms a kind of mud energy that coagulates in the outer layers and gives rise to different diseases. In the tradition of the "Guardians of Wisdom," *people were taught not only to re-program it, but also to clean it daily, by a procedure called "**flowing**" to prevent the energy from stagnating,* which can give rise to various problems mental, emotional or physical.

As it connects us with the whole Universe of energies, we can extract a filament of light from this *sphere of luminous energy* and direct it far away from our body and *will* that we come into contact *through it* with other places or beings. We can even extract information from other places or beings through these filaments. Equally, when we maintain ties of friendship with other people, beings or places, even when we are very distant from them, we remain united by these filaments of light to those people, beings or places. When we live in nature our sphere of luminous energy widens and we feel good. When we live in narrow spaces, within cities, sharing with millions of other people, this sphere of luminous energy, narrows a lot and we feel bad.

When we extract an object from some sacred place or receive something that is blessed or has beneficial power, our sphere of luminous energy feeds on the emergence of that sacred or beneficial object. When we learn to perceive with our inner eyes the luminous nature of life, we can recognize the connection we have with all life that surrounds us: stars, rivers, mountains, valleys, trees, animals, humans and other types of beings. This is also a characteristic of the level of the Condor.

CHAPTER TWENTY-ONE

The "Flowing" Drill

Your Luminous Energy Sphere is a bubble of light, or energy of "Existence," that surrounds your body, extending 3 to 6 feet in diameter around you.

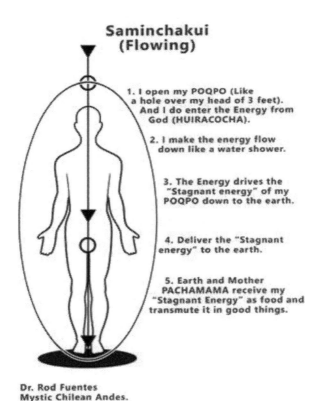

Saminchakui (Flowing)

1. I open my POQPO (Like a hole over my head of 3 feet). And I do enter the Energy from God (HUIRACOCHA).

2. I make the energy flow down like a water shower.

3. The Energy drives the "Stagnant energy" of my POQPO down to the earth.

4. Deliver the "Stagnant energy" to the earth.

5. Earth and Mother PACHAMAMA receive my "Stagnant Energy" as food and transmute it in good things.

Dr. Rod Fuentes
Mystic Chilean Andes.

Practice of Sacred Reciprocity

As if you were taking an energy shower, start by imagining a hole 3 feet in diameter opening above your head, by which the living fresh energy of the Cosmos begins to descend from God Himself. Let this energy remove, from the top to the bottom, all the stagnant energies that could be in your sphere, which produces fears, nervousness, and diseases. Imagine it washing your sphere completely.

At the same time, let it clean and strengthen the 4 levels of reality: spiritual, mental, emotional and physical. Let it flow towards the Earth and Mother Pachamama, so that it is received by Her, so that She can transmute it and give it a useful purpose. Thus, all your stagnant energy is swept away, you are freed from it, and your sphere is refreshed and cleansed of all impurity. Then you will feel the energies renewed in you, on the levels of the Condor, Hummingbird, Puma and Serpent.

You need to practice this Exercise for 5 to 10 minutes, once or twice a day, to receive all the benefits from the Exercise. (Some find it very beneficial to face the Sun to do these movements.)

This is a practice of "Sacred Reciprocity," where you receive energy from the higher, the Spiritual (God, the Divine) and you deliver it to the material Universe - the Earth and PACHAMAMA - that feeds on it, through you as an intermediary. Everything in the Andean wisdom, especially in the spiritual level of the Condor, on which everything depends, is based on the "Sacred Reciprocity." The quality of your "Reciprocity" depends on the state of your "luminous energy sphere." The more "fluid energy" you have in it, the more effective will be your "AYNI" with the Universe and other people.

The "Flowing Drill" is the essential practice to obtain a sphere of healthy, coherent and "clean" luminous energy. It will directly affect your entire being in the 4 levels of reality, and your capacity for "Sacred Reciprocity." Or, to put it another way, it affects or improves your personal power. It also affects and improves the quality of your spiritual, mental, emotional and physical health. As you cleanse your energetic body, you perfect your "Ayni," which in turn helps you climb up to the level of the Condor and the ladder of the seven steps of consciousness. This is the reason why a great teacher of the Andean tradition said, "ONLY with the Exercise of "flowing" can one reach the highest levels of consciousness and start living in the reality of the Condor."

The daily practice of "flowing" is therefore fundamental in Andean wisdom, and for your development as a human being; with this drill, you start walking the path of the "Guardians of Wisdom" of the Andes. You cannot have achievements in Andean wisdom without knowing the daily practice of "flowing" and performing it every day. It is simply a fundamental practice in the wisdom of the Andes. The "Guardians of Wisdom" of the Andes pointed out that if you "clean the stagnant energy" of your luminous energy sphere, every day, you can, over time, return to a state of "Existence," perfectly absorbent and radiant.

CHAPTER TWENTY-TWO

Exercises of Perception and Solutions

In the Four Levels of Reality

Example 1

Thing or object: Book

Perceptions at the Serpent Level: We only pay attention to the physical: number of pages, weight and size of the book.

Perceptions at the Puma Level: Thoughts occur about the author of the book and effort involved in writing the book. We may imagine the publisher, the publishing house; even the trees that must have been destroyed so that the leaves of the book could be made.

Perceptions at the Hummingbird Level: We understand the symbolic meanings of a book encompassing freedom, education, culture or progress.

Perceptions at the Condor Level: We

observe the amount of details that made this book, so that it might be in our hands today, the synchronies involved in the process, the attractive law that made the book reach those who are attuned to it by vibration. (We realize that each book has the author´s "cogito" or personal energy and consciousness within its pages.)

Example 2

Sexual Activity

Perceptions in the Serpent Level: There will only be a selfish desire for physical union, without considering anything other than the consummation of the sexual act; sex initiated only as a physical desire that will satisfy sexual desires or instinct.

Perceptions in the Puma Level: At this level, the physical desire is no longer essential or considered important. We begin to see sex as an act of, or expression of love, or as simply of pleasurable. Thoughts arise regarding responsibility, with the possibility of generating a child, and the consequences of paternity. Thoughts, also come into play with all our religious beliefs, taboos about sex or lack of them.

Perceptions at the Hummingbird Level: The sexual act is transformed into a sacred and transcendental act, that some in India and Arabia call the "Sacred Rite." This Sacred Rite is also practiced in Alchemy, where there is a transmutation and mixing of the male and female physical and energetic fluids. To achieve this chemical operation of the highest level, all the components of this alchemical operation are important and must meet certain requirements under penalty of completely failing the operation with many consequences of emotional, health, and spiritual well-being.

Perceptions in the Condor Level: Sex manifests at this level as a perfect expression of Sacred Reciprocity. Because the male function is electric and the female function is magnetic, there is an exchange of energy with their magnetic and electric counterparts, generating a perfect mixture of electromagnetic energies.

Example 3

Situation: Bad relationships with the partner and verbal aggression

Perceptions at the Serpent Level: We only pay attention to the physical which is reflected in the way we speak about our annoying partner, the gestures of our body and face when we get angry and the reactions to the words that he/she says. We respond, or maybe we flee, and then we knock on their door, it is a back and forth. To cope, we ingest an anxiolytic to calm internal tensions, or we visit the house of a relative or friend, looking for a place of greater "security." At the level of the Serpent, we depend on the instinct and do not reflect on the problems. We are functioning with the reptilian brain, that part of the brain that we share with lizards and dinosaurs, which ignore mental, emotional, creative and spiritual levels or situations.

Perceptions at the Puma Level: Thoughts occur about "why does my partner react like this, why can't we communicate better and live quieter lives?" We remember and appreciate with pleasure the good moments of our relationship and look for the causes of why this is happening now. We also question whether there is something causing these problems, an emotional pain, something from our past that makes him/her react this way. Will he/she feel sick? We question ourselves on how have we contributed to this kind of aggressive response? Will he/she need professional help? Or do we need couples' therapy to improve our relationship? At this level, we are able to perceive many more things about the situation than at the level of the Serpent; therefore, we can think of many more solutions and more efficient ones.

Perceptions at the Hummingbird Level: At this level we ask ourselves, "How can this problem become an opportunity and an advantage?" We believe that having these problems can enrich us and make us grow in many ways and can develop in us tenacity, persistence, courage, intelligence and many other things that will be valuable for our growth in the journey of our soul.

Perceptions at the Condor Level: We observe the number of causes that created these problems to be present in our relationship and analyze the type of AYNI that we are experiencing, and how to improve it in case it might get worse. We begin to repair the situation by offering more love, attention, compassion, and commitment.

IMPORTANT DRILLS TO BE PERFORMED

Exercise 1

Perception of Yourself at the Four Levels of Reality

Sit in front of a mirror. Stand approximately four to five feet from the mirror. Enter a slight twilight state of the mind without deepening it. Breathe deeply and slowly for about 5 breaths without thinking about anything as you look at your entire body or just your face. Look at the game of lights and shadows on your face and keep looking at the area between your eyebrows or the middle of your forehead, as if you were looking about 3 inches inside your skull.

At the level of the Serpent, observe how your face is simply a physical face that you know and have seen thousands of times. Do not do any kind of analysis and do not miss any judgment or emotion or feeling. Just look at the face, using the same Tratakum dynamics that you learned in the first Exercise of the Serpent level. When you have done that, now enter the level of the Puma in your perceptions going to the next level. Here continue paying attention to the eyebrows but indirectly observe the lower lines and shadows of your face, those that show your emotions, your passions, those belonging to the "animal soul" (astral body). You will now allow these emotions about yourself, the person you are currently in the world, your different roles, judgments that you make on yourself and others, to be expressed. In that slight twilight state, now keep looking as if you could explore even deeper within yourself. While you keep looking, imagine that the physical body disappears so that you can see your own astral body or "animal soul," that of emotions and passions.

It is likely that you might see forms of different animals, representing the different emotions and passions and tastes that you have dragged through several lives to the present day, or you might begin to see faces of other people, or perhaps your face disappears completely with the exception of the eyes. Remain calm, stay in the twilight state, always breathing slowly and regularly. Simply register the possible face or faces that appear. If none appear, then just pay attention to how you feel. The "luminous energy sphere" at the level of the astral body or "animal soul" contains the memories of all our previous selves.

Now rise to the level of the Hummingbird. Imagine that in addition to your physical face disappearing, your astral body also disappears so that what remains is the psyche, the human soul. You imagine that the person you are looking at in the mirror stops having a physical body and astral body to reflect what is beyond those two levels. Your physiognomy will stop changing and only one image will appear. Look carefully at the face that appears because it has a meaning and a message that is important to you at this time. Stabilize this concentrated image always in your eyebrows and allow it to reveal before you, your inner psyche, the human soul. What message does it have for you? You can also give your psyche a message that can be the same that you gave it in Exercise 1 in the chapter dedicated to the description of the level of the Hummingbird.

For example, if you are having a disease or a conflictive situation in any areas of your life, regardless of the seriousness of your condition, think about looking at yourself from the psyche level and then manifest an image of perfect health in your destiny and different futures for yourself, with health and well-being and not disharmony death or problems. This will have a tremendously powerful effect at this high level, no matter the severity of the condition. Having done this, now you indirectly look at the lines and upper shadows of your face, always looking at the center between your eyebrows, to rise to the level of the Condor. You imagine now that you stop having, not only the physical and astral body, but you also stop having the psyche; you now sensorially perceive your deepest Self, your "unconditioned being," your Immortal Divine Soul. At this level all forms dissolve in the universal energy matrix, and the only thing you will perceive is Light and Spirit.

Likewise, if you are having a disease or situation of conflict or scarcity or precariousness in any area of your life, regardless of the seriousness of your condition, when you detect your Spirit or Divine Soul as energy and Light, you send thoughts such as:

"As I am now healthy, I manifest health, well-being and perfect harmony, NOW. My Spirit is always perfect and healthy. I see only well-being, harmony and peace, I feel peace and health. I am above all disharmony, Now, Now, NOW!

To end the session, leave the twilight state, making three deep breaths and return to the ordinary consciousness.

Exercise 2

Perceptions of Another Person at the Four Levels of Reality

This is a tracking Exercise to look up information about another person in the four levels of reality. It is a deepening of Exercise 2 of the Chapter dedicated to the description of the level of the Hummingbird. It is identical to the previous one with yourself but instead of seeing yourself in a mirror, you look into the eyes of another person and check each one of his/her levels of reality or vehicles. At the Puma level you will see some of the faces in his/her past lives and the passions or emotions that govern his/her life today as well as things that must improve and be overcome.

But at the level of the Hummingbird, they stop having a physical and astral body to reflect upon and you become aware of what is beyond those two levels in his/her psyche. When you have achieved this, you can install in him/her powerful thoughts that will help him/her at that level, with all your heart. Or you can simply think that that psyche manifests the image of perfect health in its destiny and future. If you are working with a sick person, regardless of the severity of their condition, this will have a tremendously powerful effect at that level.

And finally, when you pass to the level of the Condor and the person stops having not only a physical and astral body, but also the psyche, then you will only perceive his/her deepest Self, his/her "unconditioned being" and REAL Immortal Divine Soul. At this level you send him/her thoughts such as:

"As you are healthy in your Spirit, you manifest health, well-being and perfect harmony NOW. Your Spirit is always perfect and healthy. You see well-being, harmony and peace, you feel peace and health. You are healed of all disharmony, Now, Now, NOW!

Once this is done you can tell this person, you are cured of this disease and now he/she can practice this same Exercise in the mirror where he/she will also insert at the level of the Hummingbird his/her new destiny and future of a healthy and perfect body. You can ask if they want you to continue to accompany them with thoughts to the level of the Condor. After a few months of doing this, there will be no illness or situation that might not be improved and solved at these high levels of reality.

Solving Our Problems From the Different Levels of Reality

We have already seen an example of perception and application of solutions in the four levels of reality. Now I will offer a more complete method that involves the above but suggests an additional step to choose the appropriate level in which the best solutions will be found.

Always according to the fundamental principle that states that:

> *Every problem we face must be resolved at the level at which it was created, generally, at a level higher than that in which it manifests. Because if we do it only at the level that they manifest,*
>
> *there will be a temporary solution or none at all. But from the level of the Condor EVERYTHING is healed.*

This method will also allow us to recognize at what level the situation is being caused. The application of this model includes situations of emotional mental illness, physical or economic lack, absent or bad relationships, friendship, romance and good or bad luck, etc.

The 5 stages of Solving Problems

Perception
Manifestation
Understanding
Causation
Solution or Remedy

Faced with a situation in any area of our life that brings us pain, loss or suffering, we will follow the following model of five steps:

Identify the level of reality in which it manifests:
Physical level? (Serpent)
Emotional mental level? (Puma)
Level of the psyche, superior mind or "human soul"? (Hummingbird)

Situations to be solved in our life will manifest and be caused in the first three levels only. Physical and material situations manifest from the Serpent level. Mental and emotional situations manifest from the Puma level. The psyche, superior mind or human soul issues manifest from the Hummingbird level. Suffering will never occur on the level of the Condor, because it is the level of perfection, of the Divine, of God and never contaminated or damaged in any way. Only health, perfection and healing emerge from this level. Never will some kind of imperfection manifest at this level.

Once you identified the level in which the situation, problem or disease, manifests itself, so as to understand the situation and have a complete healing vision, we will make a mental Exercise of perception and analysis in these four levels, exercising and putting in action our 4 ñawis as we have done in the previous Exercises of the book.

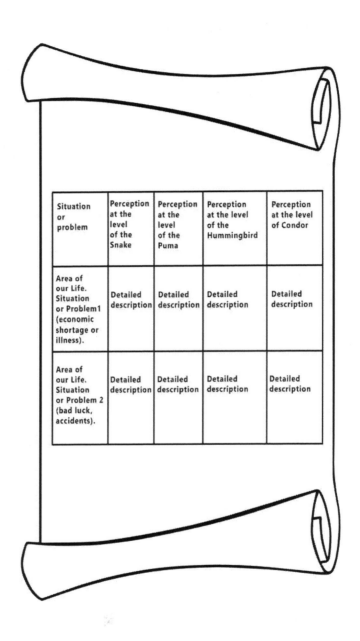

Situation or problem	Perception at the level of the Snake	Perception at the level of the Puma	Perception at the level of the Hummingbird	Perception at the level of Condor
Area of our Life. Situation or Problem1 (economic shortage or illness).	Detailed description	Detailed description	Detailed description	Detailed description
Area of our Life. Situation or Problem 2 (bad luck, accidents).	Detailed description	Detailed description	Detailed description	Detailed description

Putting into Action Our 4 Nawis

Once the situation is understood and analyzed in the 4 levels of reality and perception, we proceed to look for the level at which the problem was created, so that we can solve it successfully; keep bearing in mind the principle expressed several times in this book:

> *Every problem we face must be resolved at the level at which it was created. Generally, we look to a level higher than that in which it manifested. Because, if we do it only at the level that they manifest, there will be only a temporary solution, or none at all. But from the level of the Condor EVERYTHING is healed.*

Was this situation or problem created in the physical level? (Serpent)
Was this situation or problem created in the Emotional Mental Level? (Puma)
Was this situation or problem created at the level of the psyche or human soul? (Hummingbird)

Again, I point out that we completely discard the level of the Condor, because it is the level.

241

of perfection, of the Divine, of God, never contaminated or damaged in any way.

Therefore, from this level, things are only solved, but problems are never created.

Situations in our life will be caused in the first three levels only:

Serpent (physical material)
Puma (mental, emotional)
Hummingbird (the psyche or human soul)

It can help us to discover the level at which the situation was created in the following way:

1. Concrete: Historical tracking of how the situation began, date, age, and how it manifested from the beginning. If the cause is at the level of the psyche, it will have begun to manifest at the level of abstract thinking, imagining things, having faith or confidence that something bad would happen, or similar occurrences which gave rise to real emotions or situations in the physical world over time. The time it took, might take years, to descend from the psychic level to the mental or emotional level and then the time it took to descend from the mental emotional level to the physical one. If it started on the emotional level it simply started there with some emotional traumatic situation or *wrong mind suggestions* given by someone else, and then descended to the physical with the passage of time. This is the method of the blind man who has no eyes to see, but he can help many people to know what exists even when he is slow and imprecise.

2. Oracular: It is a method of inquiry that operates on the magical, ritualistic and level of the Hummingbird. Using the Andean altar or Misha, the "guardians of knowledge," especially the Q'eros, use three blankets to make a consecrated personal altar. One of these blankets has only two white colors to the right and black to the left. They represent duality in the Universe and "yes" or "no."

The Andean Paqo takes a small stone and passes it to the person who has the problem and asks him/her to think about giving the "identity" of that problem, situation or illness, to the stone, blowing three times over it, thinking that the problem or situation has been transferred to the stone. Later, the Paqo puts it about 30 inches above the dividing central line of the two colors of the blankets and, with both hands, asks a Yes or NO question.

For example, was this problem or situation created at the level of the person's psyche? He then lets "the charged stone" with the problem fall. If the stone falls in the white color it means yes; and if it falls in the black color it means no. Everything is done in a special Ritual environment and in my opinion, it is quite accurate. It is a method that I teach my students in the retreats when I transmit the initiations in the Andean wisdom that I received from Don Joaquín.

3. The Exercise of the dark violet room. This is a method of inquiry that operates at the level of the Condor and was mentioned with instructions on page 84. This method requires having obtained practice and certainty in the previous Exercise. Having obtained the trance state that is taught in earlier Exercises, one asks: "At what level was the problem of this or that person created?" The answers are expected and will come through an image, a phrase, or through a sense of certainty. It usually occurs through an image or phrase. If none of the methods explained here is well mastered, or there are doubts about having known the level where the problem, situation or illness was created, one simply proceeds to deal with the problem at all three levels simultaneously.

Having determined the level of cause or level of creation of the situation, proceed to step four.

4. Healing is proceeded according to the principle already discussed several times in this book.

> *Every problem we face must be resolved at the level at which it was created. Generally, to a level higher than that in which it manifests. Because if we do it only at the level that they manifest, there will be only a temporary solution or none at all. But from the level of the Condor EVERYTHING is healed.*

Some methods for healing or solution have already been explained in this book. There are many more methods that I will teach in other books or in seminars and trainings that we dictate to our students under training in the tradition of the "Guardians of Wisdom" of the Andes.

CHAPTER TWENTY-THREE

The "Guardians of Wisdom" in the Andes

Circular Time or Divine Time

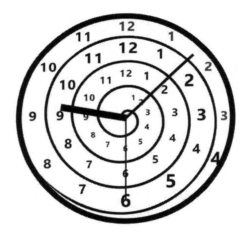

**Circular Time. Future and past are the same
word in Quenchua tongue.
If you change your future, your future
will change your present.**

Time, being a measurement of what happens in the physical world, has no existence at higher levels than the physical one; at least, time doesn´t exist as we usually understand it at the Hummingbird or the Condor levels. From the views of the Hummingbird and the Condor, to the "Guardians of Wisdom," the vision of time is completely different from that of the West, since there is no longer the idea that the effect follows the cause, and there is the concept of timelessness as well. The current view of the West is that time flows in one direction, and that the future is always before us, and the past behind, which we understand as linear time. But for the "guardians of Wisdom," time does not only advance forward like a dart blown from a blowpipe, it also rotates like a wheel, or makes the circular movement like a boomerang.

This nonlinear, or circular time, acquires a divine, or sacred character of the circle. It points out that **we can modify the present through the future and adjust events that have already occurred**. Linear time works according to the principle of cause and effect and that the past is creating the present and the present the future. For example, some people think they do not do as well in life, because they do not have the necessary education, and that's why they have economic problems in the present, which makes them unhappy. This is the concept of linear time of cause and effect on the levels of the Serpent and the Puma, which is the lowest. *In circular time, the future creates the present, and if you modify the future, which is modifiable, from the timeless and circular levels of the Condor and the Hummingbird, you can improve the present.* So, when our perception of time becomes circular, the principle is synchronicity or the synchronicity of events.

What we call *coincidence or luck is an operating principle as rigorous and exact for circular time as is causality for linear time*. The "Guardians of Wisdom" believe that the synchronous occurrence of some events, such as when we meet fortuitously with someone on the street, or watch a television show that contains a message for us, or pass a person with a sign painted on his back, this is a message for us. When crossing the street, or sitting down to drink a coffee, or listening to a special song that is playing, this calls to memory certain thoughts, and it is as significant as its cause.

Synchronicity worries about the purpose and meaning of an event, much more than the causes of it. In the concept of circular time, the future may be pushing us, or attracting us, as well as when the past pushes us forward in the concept of linear time. The reason why we do not see it this way is because our mind has been programmed to detect things and think only in a linear way. The "Guardians of Wisdom" know that the cause of a present event may, in fact, be in the future. And if unpleasant things happen, like a traffic accident that makes you late for a meeting or event, do not believe that you have bad luck, or you are an unfortunate person. It would be better for you to recognize that you are living in a circular or sacred time, and that the Universe is in your favor, attracting you from the future so as to make the events occur in the present. The bus leaves 20 minutes later because you must arrive at the destination with a certain delay to meet certain events or avoid others; it's the bus you should take, and the traffic accident allowed this to happen. In circular time the stress is reduced significantly because we now know, from the levels of the Hummingbird and the Condor, that luck or chance is part of a great rigorous plan as well.

SUPERIORITY OF DIVINE TIME

In circular time, you live in a world where you are never late or ahead, you only arrive when you arrive, and it happens that everyone also comes at the right time. This is the true concept of living in the NOW which has now been well explained or hopefully understood. I made a clock that, instead of having numbers (1, 2, 3, 4, etc.) to indicate the hours, had the word NOW instead of each of those numbers. All the time, it was NOW. Instead of saying it's 2 in the afternoon, I looked at the clock and the clock marked the time: NOW. If I looked at this watch three hours later, I again saw the correct and exact time: NOW.

Living in a Divine or Sacred time does not exempt us from our commitments, responsibilities, duties, and the need to arrive at the agreed time, but rather allows us to sustain an Ayni that we always appear at the most perfect moment. By living like this, we give the opportunity for synchronicities to occur. We thus discard the absurd idea of wanting to manipulate the world around us and "always have control" so that everything goes as planned by us. We can now solve our problems in the future, before they have even formed. We do it from the level of the Condor, so, from this level, we only need 5% of our energy to affect the world the way we want. We avoid having to occupy 95% when we leave the prison of linear time. We thus enter into the concept of timelessness, no time, where the entire Universe, including ourselves, is programming itself. Within this sacred time, we can find the most desirable future for ourselves and choose that, instead of the less desirable one that would give us more problems.

This concept has been recently incorporated by the French physicist Jean-Pierre Garnier-Malet, which he has called "temporary openings" or "unfolding of space and time." When we practice circular time, we will arrive at a destination we have chosen, instead of the one chosen for us by statistics or by the collective, whose language is those of statistics. People with a poor prognosis of disease, where statistics say they will die in the same way as other patients with the same disease, is a statistical observation. By accessing the circular time, as the French physicist Jean-Pierre Garnier-Malet points out, they can choose one of the lines of the future that leads them to a more favorable result and install that result in their future. After that, they can beat the prognosis and regain health, or have a peaceful death without pain.

Understanding the Circular Time

Infinity is a place before and after time, before the origin and after the end; this is because infinity is outside of time. Eternity, on the other hand, is a linear time concept of the concrete mind at the level of the Puma, not the Condor; it is an infinite sequence of events. *Only in infinity, you can change the events that happened in the past and change the destiny or future. In this place, the future is pushing and conditioning you as much as the past. When you get out of the time sequence, and you go into infinity, the past and the future reveal to you their keys.*

During sleep, we are not attached to matter or space. Time has no direction. It is not linear like when we dreamed of a deceased relative some time ago and at the same time you can see tomorrow and the day after tomorrow. *In circular, or divine time, the future and the past are available, to make changes in them, and everything happens at the same time.* We can only dream or imagine the world and make it come true from this timeless place, because when we raise our perception to the level of the Condor, we find it possible to experience this infinity. This a very powerful teaching I was taught by Don Joaquín on millenarian quantum Andean teachings.

The "Guardians of Wisdom" teach that if you want to change a situation, you must begin by recognizing that NOW -an extension of Infinity- IS PERFECT, and then you can begin to transform everything you want. From the Condor level -or the "quantum level of existence."

According to Isaac de Luria, the master kabbalist of the Renaissance, an infinite number of years ago, the Source of Everything, whom we call God, decided to experience Himself (Herself) and formed all the matter of the Universe. So, each of His manifestations possessed the divine qualities of omnipresence and omniscience. His divine nature had to be set apart from them. Therefore, he created a kind of vacuum and retired away from them to make possible for these manifestations to exist, in order to successfully know Himself through them. But, still these material things and beings - especially humans- had His (Her) existence in them. When we live in linear time, with the object of living life in a material world governed by the clock, we lose that divine essence; this is what people who are trapped in physical matter and the collective unconscious mind expect. But when we step out of linear time and experience timelessness, and circular time, we reclaim right away our deified nature and begin to remember who we truly are, as legitimate extensions of God Himself. In linear time, governed by the clock, we are forgetting, in daily life, that we possess the characteristics of God. We fall into a dream and an illusory world. Instead of thinking at the level of the Condor, which is what we should have done, we become victims of events, instead of being lords and owners of them, as is incumbent upon those who possess the divine nature. In circular time, on the contrary, everything we do will obtain a sacred character; even if we are brushing our teeth, we lose ourselves in that wonderful, sacred, moment, of NOW.

"When I was a child the Idea of a God that had no beginning or no end tormented me day and night. How could something or SOMEONE exist who had never been created? This question shook me and made me feel completely-literally-dizzy. But I found solace and comfort, and my mind came to peace, when Don Joaquín explained to me the concept of circular time. God lived in circular time. And I was living in a material world, with my mind in linear time; that's why I was mentally tormented and couldn't understand

Him. I was limiting Him with my restricted thought. I immediately understood that if I began to live in circular time I would become as Him.

Therefore, instead of waiting to recover our divine nature and return to paradise, someday or after death, *the "Guardians of Wisdom" point out that HERE in the material world and NOW is the ideal time and place to enter there and recover our divine, or heavenly essence, and make a heaven on Earth.*

That's one of the most important lessons, step number one, we teach our students in our trainings on millenarian quantum Andean teachings.

CHAPTER TWENTY-FOUR

The Temples in The Andes

Due to being in a special archaeo-astronomical location, the ancient temples of the Andes are still places of "power," that contain stored energy sources, able to produce a tremendous inner awakening in the human being. The Andes are monuments of energetic activity of great potential and are places carefully designed to start the transformation of your being and reset your mind.

Purposes of the Temples in the Wisdom of the Andes

In the ancient temples of the Andes, what was sought, was to awaken and free human beings from everything that enslaved them and allow them to advance through their own development. It was a place that allowed them to achieve a reconditioning of all their limitations, to lead them to reach first their happiness as a human being, and then help them to rise to their highest potential with different degrees of realization. Contrary to what has happened in other later religious temples of the West and East, where the objective has been to control and dominate by dogma and fanaticism, Andean wisdom aimed to liberate.

The opposite of many later religions, which spoke of "dying to be happy," or "suffering to gain salvation," *in the Andes, there was always talk of connecting with the abundant creative energy of the Earth, of the mountains and God, so as to have fulfillment in everything, right now.* They sought freedom from scarcity and pain by giving conscious existence to abundance and eliminated scarcity by taking away its existence.

These are powerful keys of the teachings of the Andes that are contained in their "Andean codes" and in the 4 levels of reality and perception of reality that these "Guardians of Wisdom" have transmitted to us. *The teachings of Andean wisdom are meant to help people find heaven here, while living on the Earth and to stop expecting to find happiness only in the afterlife.* Their goal was to awaken awareness to these deep truths and not to continue deceiving people or being deceived by others. Some very advanced knowledge in the Andes was protected, and guarded tenaciously only for those who, after having advanced, were ready to be trained to receive it. The most advanced of this "private" knowledge in the

Andes is like a key, or a code, and that key is not passed on to those who you do not know well, neither to those who do not know themselves. These keys also have the power to open dimensions, or higher levels of reality, which can seem madness to those who live enslaved to the material world, spiritually and mentally asleep, and clinging to dogmas and false doctrines.

Three Main Temples and their Presence in the Andes of Bolivia and Chile Today

The ancient Temples of the Andes, that date back at least 10,000 years, were very different from our current churches. They were truly foci and places of the transformation of human consciousness, for the transcendence of the human being and the achievement of lasting happiness. Some, like the Temple of the Serpent, were dedicated to medicine and to the physical; others, like the Temple of the Condor, were dedicated to love and Ayni; and others, to the different cerebral and spiritual centers within us.

A few, like those of the Puma, were *fully focused on the subconscious reconditioning, which is one of the first objectives* that enables the achievement of human happiness. Some of the tools that make this work possible have been described in the initial pages of this book. Work on the subconscious was shared between the Temples of the Serpent and the Puma, because the subconscious mind is linked to both the instincts (Serpent) and the emotions (Puma). The "Guardians of Wisdom" pointed out that the part of the subconscious related to the most instinctive and "organic," physical part of the human being, was like a Serpent, the anaconda or South American boa, which is known as "AMARU," which can strangle with great ease any large animal or adult person. But when it is domesticated, it can become the "guardian" of the home and be left even to the care and protection of the family, as it is today in certain areas of the Amazon.

Each one of the ancient temples in the millenary Andes corresponded to very specific themes, to work for the perfection of the human being and his/her happiness. The temples were dedicated to the awakening of the human being. They were generally inserted in the middle of nature in the vicinity of a mountain. They were also located on a mountain or hill in the vicinity of running water or a water source, within a cavern or grotto, or near a natural phenomenon of nature. They contained within them an Andean cross, called "CHAKANA," that was a representation of the stars of the Southern Cross in the heavens. In addition, they are usually aligned to some beneficial constellations of heaven and were special places of instruction.

Today, the temples of religions are places to control people and have them put to sleep under certain dogmas or ideas, from which they cannot escape at the level of the Puma alone. They would become subjects to the authority of one man, or several men. This was not taught by the ancient priesthood whose temples were designed to **free man from men**. In this way, we can see that "the teachings of the Andes" were not a religion." It does not conform to the modern concept that has been made of this word, because they dealt with the awakening of the being and his happiness here on Earth, and not in the beyond. It could be religion in the sense of re-linking or re-uniting the person to the Apus (Sacred Beings of the mountains in charge of the spiritual evolution of human beings), or to Pachamama, the mother of everything, and to God, Huiracocha, the Source of all. But it does not conform to the concept of religion that people have in their minds when thinking about any of the religions of the world today with their set of dogmas and beliefs that they inculcate in their parishioners and churches.

Modern religions are a set of dogmatic ideas and doctrines that are used to control people and not allow them to assume or awaken the inner God, which is something very different from what the tradition of the Andes did for more than 10,000 years. We see many people who are affiliated with spiritual groups, religions, or personal development cults, whose life was made worse. They are trapped by the illusion of time, always busy, always in a hurry, full of external worries and distractions, without knowing anything about themselves. In the Andes, for thousands of years, people have identified themselves with living with divinity in the mountains, in nature where Pachamama lives, and with the Sacred Apus or spiritual beings of the mountains. In the Andes, all of nature was considered a great temple.

The wisdom and knowledge of the Andes indicates that there is agreement and harmony between the constellations of the sky, the stars, and the things below, like the mountains, the valleys, the geographical features, and the temples below, that were built by the ancient "Guardians of Wisdom" or Andean priests or Paqos of the past. In the traditions of the Andes, the Earth was a mirror of the sky above. The first thing that had to take place was a healthy balance between the masculine and the feminine. The ancient peoples of the East called this duality, where there may be conflict, but in the Andes, it was called "duality in harmony" (<u>Yanantin</u> in the Quechua tongue).

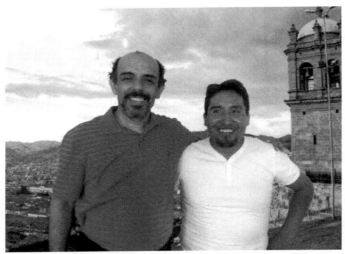

Here Dr. Rod Fuentes is pictured with Nicolás Pauccar, who stars in the movie "Humano." Humano is a documentary that narrates the journey of a young man into the Andes mountains where he learns to discover the origin of man.

CHAPTER TWENTY-FIVE

"Guardians of Wisdom" Versus

Shamans' Drug Use for Spiritual Development

The "Guardians of Wisdom," Paqos, among whom are also the Q'eros, have **never** called themselves **shamans**. They call themselves "**Andean Priests**" or Paqos, a word which means **priest** and "reborn" healer. They dislike it when you call them shamans because they consider it a kind of insult to them. In order for Westerners to understand and categorize the word 'Paqo,' which is something new for them, these "Guardians of Wisdom," or Andean priests and priestess, have been **erroneously** called "**shamans.**" Most people in Western society think that a priest is someone who prays or teaches in a church. But Andean priests and priestesses walk in contact with nature, as shamans do, having a close relationship with the world of "*living energies*" and the multiple beings of nature and the Universe. That´s also why they have been confused by Westerners with shamans.

The differences between a shaman and an Andean priest or "Paqo" is as great as the difference between a horse and a zebra. *A shaman is someone who uses herbal medicines and drugs to go into a trance and travel in the spiritual world.* The shaman *has no formal training* as an Andean priest or Paqo from the "guardians of the wisdom." The "guardian of wisdom" or Paqos, respect all traditions, including the Amazon shamans, but they *do not use any type of drugs*. They *do not need drugs to work with the living energy* or to travel through the dimensions that surround us or within us. They learned to Exercise their spiritual abilities through years and years of training in the Andean schools, and learned about the deep knowledge of healing, and the "luminous energy sphere" that contains the codes of existence.

A shaman is someone who has self-made himself/herself as a shaman, and in most cases, the shaman has never had a master who trained them. Sometimes they were psychics who came in touch with the spirits of nature or the plants in the jungle and they learned from those spirits the nature and powers of the plants; many times, using drugs from those same plants for certain purposes.

On the other hand, the Andean priest or Paqo, through the work of "living energy," transformed their past to consciously leave linear time and enter circular time. In this place, they reconnect with their original essence and begin their spiritual journey. Andean priests and priestesses or Paqos, among whom today are also many Westerners, such as the author of this book, have trained their minds, to awaken the dormant brain centers and the ñawis (spiritual eyes), which are at the highest level of the Hummingbird and Puma centers, normally asleep in people. Along with this, they "weaved" the power belts in their "luminous energy spheres" that surround their physical body.

The "Guardians of Wisdom" or Paqos are descendants of the Inca priesthood, the shamans are instead descended through tribal traditions. Shamans who have not been trained, *need and depend on substances to access these spiritual realities*. I consider it very important to stop here and make a clarification about the drugs used by the shamans of the tribes of the Amazons.

Many Westerners think that the drugs used by shamans are equivalent to the hallucinogens or stimulants used in the West. I refer to the drugs used for fun or indulging in drugs that make you have a "good time." This is the classic image of a group of hippies enjoying a good party with their friends, using

LSD, cocaine, heroin, methamphetamines or marijuana, to have fun, relax or stimulate themselves. The truth is completely different. The drugs that the shamans of the South American jungle use are considered *"sacred plants" that must be treated with great respect by the shaman and those who consume them as medicine.* Its ingestion leads the person to have a very powerful and strong experience, often a painful and agonizing experience, which must be carefully watched by an expert. The best-known drug is the Ayahuasca and secondarily the Wachuma or "Hierba de San Pedro" (Saint Peter Cactus).

The Ayahuasca takes a person to an experience similar to physical death. Those who consume it observe passing in front of their mental eyes all their life; this is also reported to happen with those who live the experience of death, they report having seen their whole life pass in front of them in the smallest details, because they are accessing the unconscious data base that has all the records of past experiences. In some cases, Ayahuasca also produces a series of rather unpleasant physical symptoms such as vomiting and diarrhea. This is because it is a true purge of traumas from the past, energies and emotions stagnant for years within the "luminous energy sphere" of a person. And for that reason, its consumption I only recommend as a support for a psychological treatment in the case of addictions, alcoholism, very intense depression, or psychosomatic illnesses. It is a valuable tool for these cases and under the guidance of an Ayahuasca expert and always accompanied by a psychologist or psychotherapist; in these cases, I have seen good results.

I personally treat many cases of addictions, depression, and alcoholism, with "Reconditioning of the Subconscious Mind" (RSM). And, I do recommend the use of Ayahuasca to some of my patients under the care of an expert and the support of a psychologist in the situations already mentioned, but only when dealing with severe addictions, to those that come to me to be healed. The final words on Ayahuasca will be found at the end of this book.

On the subject of shamanism in this book, these drugs have a history of being used exclusively for cultural purposes. To clarify, to those who make the great mistake of confusing an Andean priest, "guardian of the wisdom," with a shaman of the jungle; this is a confusion that has become very common and has occurred most of the time accidentally, or simply by misinformation. But in other cases, it has been purposely and commercially carried out by unscrupulous Westerners who, living far from South America or the Andes, have purposely tried to confuse the people of the United States and Europe, with the sole purpose of confusing and profiting from this idea.

I was born in the Chilean Andes Mountains, just kilometers from where the great Incas, more than 500 years ago, regularly spent two years of vacation. And even though my parents are of Spanish European descent, and my education was wholly given in the formation of a Westerner, I lived in the middle of the Andes and had contact with the ancestral practices of both "Guardians of Wisdom," and Mapuches (Chilean shamans). From my earliest childhood, I heard mentioned in my European-style home, terms such as Andean "despachos," (Andean offerings to Pachamama and the Holy Apus) "living energy," ancestral herbs, Inca herbs, "personal energy transmission," and "magic." And also, since childhood I heard a lot about the healings carried out both by Mapuches and shamans with well-known people of my family and in myself with certain diseases that I suffered as a little child. I have lived most of my life in the middle of the Andes mountain in Chile, where my own family have extensive lands in the

Andes mountains, in the territory that was part of the ancient Incan Empire, and that today is being completely rediscovered by archaeologists.

Growing up under the influences of the Andean mountains, at the early age of 14, I was initiated into the 7 Sacred Rites of the Andes. Most of the teachings I am sharing here in this book, by an Andean teacher "guardian of the wisdom", Paqo and priest, Don Joaquín Freire, from the Rari Mountains, Chile. And never in the Andean priesthood did I hear about the use of drugs or similar substances that were necessary for the internal or spiritual development of the future Paqo. I have only seen administering or suggesting the herb of San Pedro (Wachuma), by an Andean Paqo or "guardian of wisdom." The people that were given Wachuma were great intellectuals, who had a hard time having perceptions through the ñawi at the level of the Hummingbird, or at the level of the psyche. They needed Wachuma for that specific purpose, to open their mental eyes to higher realities, as an external help, and only once or twice in their life.

Today I continue to live in the middle of the Andes Mountains under the influence of the Sacred Apus (Holy beings of the mountains) and in the proximity of the most powerful Inca temples of my nation, such as the temple of the Serpent AMARU (Hue-ten or "Santa Lucía" Hill) and I can say with full authority that the *Andean wisdom and drugs are things completely independent one from the other.* And I finish here talking about these substances, drugs or shamans of the jungle, because they have nothing to do with the valuable substance of this book, except to clear up the great confusion and ignorance that exists in the minds of many Westerners, especially in the USA where this book is going to be launched.

In this book we are dealing with the Andean priesthood, who are the "keepers and guardians of knowledge and wisdom" of the Andes. These initiates and masters of the "living energy", are the direct descendants of the imperial priesthood of the royal house of the Incas of the past. They have in their custody the secret of the Andes for almost 500 years after the destruction of the Incan empire at the hands of the Spaniards. The word 'Paqo' is Quechua (the native language of the Inca) and comes from the word Paqocha, which is the "newborn" alpaca colt. He/she is born in the world completely pure, innocent and with the softest wool when they take their first steps in the world. The Paqos struggle to walk in this world like a newborn baby, or an alpaca colt, that without fear sees the world through the heart with purity, softness and joy. Calling yourself Paqo "guardian of the wisdom" of the Andes, means walking in the tradition of the Inca Paqos as a guardian of the *"Universe of living energy,"* which includes the Earth and the worlds that are at our side. It means walking as a wise man/woman, healer and servant of the Earth, with this medicine of authentic and pure energy, which has passed from Paqo to student for thousands of years in the mountains of the Andes of Colombia, Ecuador, Peru, Bolivia, Argentina and Chile.

Becoming a Paqo and more importantly yet, for the establishment of the New Era, is becoming a "Chaca Runa", a "citizen bridge." A Western "citizen bridge" is one who integrates the wisdom and knowledge of the West with the wisdom and traditions of the Andes, as has the author of this book. This means developing all that is contained in this book and receiving the three main initiations to awaken deep healing and transformation with your relationship with the Universe by unlocking the three centers of power in a human being. Integrating all this into the middle of a Westerner's life, with your daily life among people and friends, is your practice.

You will begin to control and heal with energy and change situations within your life and that of others, and become a powerful agent for the New Era, and the fulfillment of the Andean prophecy.

CHAPTER TWENTY-SIX

What Do You Think of The Future?

Among those who find the history and mysticism of the Andes of interest, it is widely reported that when the Spaniards conquered the Incas, nearly 500 years ago, the last Pachacuti, or great change, took place. The "Guardians of Wisdom," among them, the Q'eros, have been waiting for the next Pachacuti to take place; when the things that were upside down will fall back into its right place and order emerges from chaos again.

During the last five centuries, the "Guardians of Wisdom" kept its sacred knowledge well protected, until the end. In recent years, the signs that the great moment of change that was to come were fulfilled - "the lagoons of the high mountains dried up, the condor became almost extinct, and the Golden Temple was discovered, after the great earthquake of 1949 that represented the wrath of the Sun."

The prophecies are not all doom and gloom, there is optimism. Even though these prophecies refer to the end of time as we understand it, it is an end of a wrong way of thinking, being and relating to nature and the

Earth. In the coming years the "Guardians of Wisdom" hope that we will arise again during a golden age, a golden millennium of peace.

The prophecies also allude to several tumultuous changes on Earth and in our psyche, allowing us to redefine and improve our relationships with nature and with our own spirituality. This is ratified by the great global challenges that the Earth is experiencing, in the moments that I write this, including the melting of the poles, floods, droughts, water scarcity, extensive earthquakes, tsunamis, population migrations, climate change, change of the magnetic poles of the Earth, pollution of the oceans and possible change of the terrestrial axis. These are things that are usually heard today in everyday conversation and in the media. All of the above will obviously become even more serious and life on the planet will become very difficult, making an extreme situation for the human race and civilization as we now know it.

The next Pachacuti, or "great change", which the "Guardians of Wisdom" have been waiting for almost 500 years has already begun, and after this tumultuous world change, a new human being will emerge, but only after a period of great confusion. According to the "Guardians of Wisdom" among whom we also count some Q'eros, the chaos and confusion characteristic of this period will last several years. The paradigm of European civilization will continue to collapse day by day and the actions of the peoples of Earth will react as a devastating boomerang that is forced on themselves. More importantly, the leaders of the "Guardians of Wisdom" speak of a tear in the very fabric of time. This offers us the opportunity to describe ourselves not as what we have been in the past, both personally and collectively, but as what we will become.

Pachacuti also refers to a great Inca chief who lived at the end of the fourteenth century. It is said that he built Machu Picchu, and that he was the architect of an empire of equal size to the United States. For the Incas, Pachacuti was a spiritual prototype, a Master, a luminous being out of time. He was a Messiah, but not in the Christian sense, of being the only Son of God. On the contrary, he is considered as a symbol and a promise of what we can become in these coming times. He personifies the essence of the prophecies of the Pachacuti, since "Pacha" means "Earth", or "time", and "Cuti" means "to put back or putting things in their place." His name also means "transformer of the Earth."

The prophecies of the Pachacuti are well known in the Andes. There are those in the Andes who believe that the prophecies refer to the return of the Pachacuti Inca chief to defeat those who usurped the land of the Incas. But this is not the case, for the Andean priests, the return of Pachacuti is taking place collectively. It is not the return of a single individual, instead, it means what we are becoming as a human species, the global consciousness. It is an emergency process that concerns all the peoples of the entire world and not to a particular nation or empire.

*The material in this chapter on the Pachacuti prophesy is mostly derived from the author's time spent with professor of archaeology and Paquo, Dr. Juan Núñez del Prado, the son of Oscar Núñez del Prado, who led the first expedition high up into the Andes mountains, to the "guardians of knowledge."

CHAPTER TWENTY-SEVEN

The Karpays - The Seven Sacred Rites of The Andes

The "Guardians of Wisdom" have served as the keepers of the rites and prophecies of their Inca ancestors. Prophecies are useless unless one has the keys. The Andean Karpay (initiation rites) plant the seed of knowledge, or the seed of Pachacuti, in the "luminous energy sphere" of the person who receives the initiation. It is up to each person to water and care for that seed so that it grows and flourishes and gives birth to a healthy plant or a tree. The rites are only a transmission of potential. The Karpays connect the person with an old lineage of knowledge and power that the individual cannot access by himself and needs the help of that lineage. Ultimately, this power can provide the impetus for a person to take a leap and become an Inca, a Luminous Being. From that moment, that person will be directly related to the stars, the cosmos, the Universe of "living energy" and all beings, like the Inca Sun of cosmology; it's about recovering our luminous nature.

The "Guardians of Wisdom" believe that we must destroy the old self, along with the old models of spirituality and philosophies that have not worked in the past, and go through the rites of self-renewal, thus becoming a kind of midwife of a new way of thinking. We need to demystify what we have not understood and learn to honor and respect our Mother Pachamama, the Earth and our Father God, as well as the Sun and the heavens, and learn from everyone and everything around us.

The "Guardians of Wisdom" believe that the doors between the worlds are opening again, and there are holes in time that are becoming available for us. We can go through them and enter into the great beyond, where we can explore our extraordinary human capacities. The recovery of our luminous nature is today a possibility for all those who dare to take the leap. The "Guardians of Wisdom" do not have a Buddha or a Christ to follow. Rather they say: "Follow your own path, learn from the rivers, the trees and rocks, honor the Christ, the Buddha, your brothers and sisters, honor Mother Earth and the Source of Everything, honor yourself and all creation. Look with the eyes of your soul and commit yourself to the essentials." These are the teachings of the Andes to which this book is dedicated.

CHAPTER TWENTY-EIGHT

Last Words About "Ayahuasca"

The reference I have made in the title of this book and also in the first pages of it, to the "master plants" such as Ayahuasca, and to the mistakes in the minds of misinformed people believing that this plant could confer upon them spiritual development, must be given serious attention. Their real use, their true purpose, and worthiness as medicine, has been exclusively to clarify things and spare people a lot of expenses and suffering as a result of looking for something in a place where it does not exist. Another huge mistake made by many people is the false belief of Ayahuasca supporting spiritual development and confusing an Andean priest, guardian of wisdom, or descendant of the Imperial House of the Incas, with a shaman or man of the jungle.

There is a confusion too common among the masses that has occurred most of the time accidentally, or simply by misinformation, that there are no differences between an Inca priest and an Inca shaman. It is the same false belief, that occurs in the consuming of Ayahuasca as well. This has been purposely and commercially carried out by unscrupulous Westerners, who, living far from South America or the Andes, have purposely created this confusion in the United States and Europe, with the sole purpose of profiting somehow or in some way from these false ideas.

Addressing Andean Priests and Guardians of Wisdom, or "Paqos, in the Andes and "Shamans" in the Amazon

The Andean priests among whom are also most of the Q'eros have **never** called themselves **shamans**. They call themselves "**Andean Priests**" or Paqos, which means "reborn" healer. Sometimes they are called "Guardians of Wisdom" in the Andes Mountains. They dislike very much when you call them shamans because they have never been shamans.

In order for Westerners to understand and categorize the word 'Paqo', Andean priest, or "Guardians of Wisdom," which is something too new for them to understand, they **very erroneously** and improperly call the Andean

Priests as **"shamans."** Also, because most people in Western society think that a priest is someone who prays or preaches in a church, they have identified with their definitions and mistakenly labeled Andean Priests with these Western definitions. Andean priests and Guardians of Wisdom in the Andes Mountains, walk also in contact with nature, as shamans do, and also have a close relationship with the world of "*living energies,*" the Kawsay, the first Andean Code in this book, and the multiple beings of nature and the Universe; these similarities are why they have been confused by Westerners with shamans. The differences between a shaman and an Andean "Paqo" are great indeed.

A *shaman* is someone who normally uses herbal medicines and "*master plants*" (not Ayahuasca, that is a death experience with many unpleasant symptoms, but others such as "Saint Peter Cactus") to go into a trance and travel in the spiritual world. This is because the shaman *has no formal training* as an Andean priest, Paqo, or guardian of wisdom and need these substances to "take heaven by force."

Paqos, or Guardians of Wisdom, respect all traditions, including the Amazon shaman, but *do not use any type of substance to get or speed their spiritual vision*. They *do not need substances to work with the living energy* or to travel through the dimensions that surround us or within us. They learned to Exercise their spiritual abilities through years and years of training in the Andean schools of wisdom and acquire deep knowledge about healing and the "luminous energy field" that contains the code of existence in all human beings.

A shaman is someone who is self-made as a shaman and most of the time has never been trained by a master or teacher and they have never had formal training as a Paqo. Sometimes they were psychics living in the jungle who came in touch with the spirits of nature, or the plants, and they learned from those spirits of the plants how to heal or achieve a deep trance. On the other hand, the Guardians of Wisdom, Andean priest or Paqo, through the work of "living energy," have transformed their past to consciously leave linear time and enter circular time, which is called the Divine time. In this place, they reconnected with their original essence and began their spiritual journey.

Paqos, among which today are also many Westerners such as the author of this book, have trained their minds, brains, and Spirit to awaken the sleeping centers, the ñawis, or different centers of perception. Along with this, they "weaved" their power belts in the "luminous energy field." The Paqos, or Guardians of Wisdom in the Andes, are descendants of the Inca priesthood, the Royal House of the ancient Inca, and before them the inhabitants of the lost island of "MU." The shamans are, instead, tribal and live in the jungle. Shamans who have not been trained by spiritually Illuminated Masters, therefore **need and depend on substances to access these spiritual realities**, otherwise they are unable, at will, to achieve any level of spiritual awakenings.

I have, previously in this book, made an important clarification that was also given to me by a great guardian of wisdom in the Andes when I began the Andean path. He warned me about the "master plants" used by the shamans of the tribes of the Amazons. Another great mistake is that many Westerners think that the substances used by shamans are equivalent to the hallucinogens or stimulants used in the West. I refer to drugs for pleasurable experiences or the indulging in drugs that make you have a "good time." This is the classic image of a group of hippies enjoying a good party with their friends, using LSD, cocaine, heroin, methamphetamines or marijuana, to have fun, relax or stimulate themselves.

The truth is completely different. As I explained before, these sacred or "master plants" have great medicinal purposes, are able to heal a lot of illnesses that are a nightmare for modern Western medicine and must be treated with great respect and be used only by a good qualified healer and expert. They are never to be confused as a means to reach illumination or spiritual development, because it has never been used for that purpose. None of the true and legitimate Guardians of Wisdom in the Andes have ever suggested the use of these plants for Enlightenment or for permanent acquisitions of psychic abilities.

CHAPTER TWENTY-NINE

The Way of the Heart

Paqos- Healers of the Andes

The "Guardians of Wisdom" call the tradition of the Andes "The Way of the Heart," since it is based on beauty, humility and compassion. The Paqos are known in the Andes as healers, teachers and guides. They walk as their own healers in contact with the sacred forces of "living energy," the Universe, the Mountains and the Earth (Pachamama). It is a journey from the soul to the heart, and a path of service for others; to help, heal and share with everyone. It's about helping ourselves and helping the planet from within and following our dreams. To walk the path of a "Paqo," is to help oneself and others to open up to all the gifts that we carry within ourselves, and to make us return to a deep contact with the "*living energies*" of the Universe and of the Earth; to walk again as a child of the Sun and the Earth (Pachamama). It is time to learn to walk with one foot in the spirit world and the other foot in the physical and material world. We must communicate completely with the *living energy* in the Universe through our soul, Spirit, and through our physical altar; which in the Andes is called "Misha."

The "Misha" is a personal package of physical, emotional, mental and spiritual healing, symbolically representing the Universe, and is a main tool that some Paqos use in their journey to their destination which allows them to help others. Through this altar, or "Misha," various cures are achieved for themselves, and for their peers and a balance is found for all situations of imbalance that they find on their path of service to humanity. The "Misha" physically contains healing stones, that in the Andes are called "cuyas" (being charged with affections), and other elements of "personal energy," that when joined together form an energetic tool of physical, mental, emotional and spiritual healing. The healing stones and the objects they encounter during their journey through life are collected for this "Misha" or personal altar, that allows some "Guardians of Wisdom" to maintain a powerful awareness of their past constantly on their mind.

For their growth as a people, the objects that are gathered are gifts from the Earth or the Universe that they pick up on their path as priests. They are linked by filaments of light, or "*living energy,*" to the places where certain spiritual experiences or personal growth were lived by them.

The "Paqo" lives with the beings of nature, and when one finds the right balance, these beings help in the work of healing yourself; they also help you to walk your own path in the land of service to others. It is a work of love. The "Paqo" is using the energy of nature and the universal forces to heal the wounds of his past, and those of others, to fully enter into a deep relationship with the Mother PACHAMAMA who has sustained him throughout his lives. These Guardians walk on this planet as *keepers of the Earth*, as administrators of an ancient medicine. A new vibration has been felt again, starting in the year 2007.

This healing power, in the Inca tradition, is the ability to listen and communicate with the flow of *living energy* that is the cornerstone in everything you see around you. When you start to do this, you will be able to direct this energy with your mind, soul and spirit towards beneficial purposes, such as the healing of the personal physical, mental, affectional, and financial well-being. Personal power, therefore, consists in consciously traveling between the 3 worlds or realities of "*living energy,*" and receiving and giving ancient rites and initiations from the warmth and refuge of the sacred mountains of the Andes. The "Paqos" have been rooted in the healing traditions of the Andes mountains of Colombia, Ecuador, Peru, Bolivia, Argentina and Chile for thousands of years. They represent powerful values such as: balance, impeccability, reciprocity, love, wisdom, integrity and discipline.

Although the tradition is taken in an incredibly serious way, the joy and laughter of the soul and the spirit are not lost for any reason. A Paqo realizes that life is not personal, but that everything is happening for us and not against us. It does not snow to cool us, it just snows. But if we are unbalanced, the Universe will show us, creating life situations that tell us who we are and give us the opportunity to get out of this imbalance. The "Guardians of Wisdom" see the opportunities in each place, listen to the call of their soul and their spirit, and they also follow their dreams to make them manifest in their lives.

All Westerners who were not born in the Andes and who do not live in the Andes, now have the opportunity to receive training as "Guardians of Wisdom" or Andean Paqos. You can represent this beautiful universal tradition that has come into force through the prophecy of 2007 as well, and combine it fully with your

Western personal, religious and academic beliefs, as the author of this book has done. The author of this book, even though he lives in the mountains of the Chilean Andes, is a man of science who combines his scientific knowledge with the Andean tradition. He firmly keeps his beliefs linked to the Andean tradition, just as the Incas of the past have done.

This prophecy has said that the time belongs now to the Westerners, that they are the ones who have harmed the earth and must repair it, not only physically, but more importantly, from the energetic and the spiritual. They must combine the ancient traditions of the "Guardians of Wisdom" with the knowledge of the modern scientific world.

The prophecy clearly states that ...

"The Condor (the Andean tradition) and the Eagle (the knowledge of the Western world) will fly together."

And when this happens, we will be living in a New Era, completely different from the old and decadent one that we have known.

The prophecy for these times is that the Condor and the Eagle will fly together, and that is what will lead humanity to a "Luminous Age."

Prophecy does not speak of teaching only the Andean tradition, because, like any other, including the Vedic, esoteric, Buddhist, Christian, Kabbalistic, or Jewish philosophy, it does not have the full power to lead Westerners to a New Era. The main thing that this power has is the combination of the "wisdom of the Andes" with the wisdom and knowledge of the West. That is what will produce the true Magic for the change in humanity. Such a task is not in the hands of the Qeros, "Guardians of Wisdom," or the indigenous Paqos of Peru, Colombia, Ecuador or Chile, but with the Westerners who have been instructed in both traditions. Those that are called "Chaka runas" or "citizen bridges," are required to fulfill this prophecy. These "Chaka runas," who have been properly instructed in the fourth level of consciousness, are the catalyst for the beginning of the "Age of the Condor and Eagle."

The fourth level of consciousness allows a human being to combine, without contradictions and without confusion, two seemingly different philosophical or religious traditions. It is an impossible task for those who have not reached this level. This book was written by a Westerner who has been thoroughly trained in Western and Andean philosophy and knowledge. Therefore, he is properly prepared as a "Chana Runa" or citizen bridge" who has also been trained in the "Qanchis Pata Ñan" or "ladder of the 7 rungs of consciousness".

GLOSSARY of Quecha Words

ANAQ PACHA – The Celestial World; the world of Huiracocha, Wiracocha, God.

ANDEAN KARPAY – initiation rites

APU - Lord or Superior One; Superior Spiritual Hierarchy; Spirit Lord of Ausantage in Peru

APUKUNAS - other Spiritual Beings that live around the world

APUS - Holy Ones who inhabit the Holy Mountains; Sacred Spirits of the Mountains who live in the Light and are in charge of human beings.

ANYA – Andean Code for Reality Platforms; understanding these helps you to understand all viewpoints.

AYNI - RECIPROCITY 1st Code Andean Codes; AYNI is always practice full of Love with the Holy Beings

AYNI - Rite of the harmonic balance or RECIPROCITY

AYNI – the universal law of the cosmos like Golden Rule, do unto others as you would have done to you

AYNI INAIKUCH IS - Live in Ayni

CHAKANA – an Andean cross that is a representation of the stars of the Southern Cross in the heavens

CHANA RUNA – Citizen bridge

CHUMPIS - Energetic Belt

CURANDERO – Healer

CUTI – to put back or to put things in their place

DESPACHOS - gifts given to Pachamama

Don Joaquin Freire - Inca Master of Rari Mts. Chile who taught Humberto the 7 Rites of Andes

HAMPI - Rite of the Healer

HANAQ PACHA – Upper world

HAWEYS - special gifts given to Pachamama; Haweys dispatch/petition through devotion of reciprocity

HOMO LUMINOUS - being filled with Light

HUCHA - Heavy Energy

HUIRACOCHA - Our Spiritual Father

IACHEY – Andean Code To Know; Wisdom

INCA MUJU - Immortal Soul

INCA MUJU - Seed of Light; Spark or Particle of God; Drop of Wiracocha

JOHAY – your Poqpo or personal energy sphere is also the vehicle for the unconscious/subconscious body and like a computer has registered codes of energy or memories of your youth.

KARPAY - Spiritual Initiation; living energy or living energy of God

KAWSAY PACHA – Andean Code for Existence

KAWSAY PUIRY - consciously walking down the path of living energy of spirituality

KUNA – designates as plural

LLANKEY – Andean Code for Dare/Work; pronounced YANKAY

Mama Allpa - Mother Earth

MAMA ALLPA - Planet Earth

MAMA KILLA - Mother Moon

MAMA UNU - Mother Water

MAMACHA - Holy Mother; Universal or Sacred Mother; MOTHER MARY

MANQUEHUE – "the place of God"

MISHA – Andean altar

MAPUCHES – Chilean shamans

MOSOK - Rite of the custodian of the sacred energy of the stars or energy from the upper world

MUNAY – Andean Code for Love; message of Love subject to conscious choice; combination of Love, Desire, Will mixed in one divine force for good

NAWI - Spiritual Eyes

NAWPA - means indistinctly, past and future

PACHA – Earth or Time

PACHACUTI – Great Inca chief who lived at the end of the Fourteenth Century; it is said that he built Machu Picchu; a spiritual prototype; a luminous being out of time. Since "Pacha" means Earth or Time and "Cuti" means to put back or put things in their place, his name also means "transformer of the Earth.

PACHAMAMA - Mother;" Mother time-space;" matter; actually, refers to the <u>unlimited universal quantum field in the three times.</u>

PAQOCHA – "newborn" alpaca colt

PAQOS - Andean Priest or Priestess

PEDRO de VALDIVIA - Spanish Conqueror

PHANA Tradition of the Andean Mysticism rep. by Don Benito Qorihuaman of Qosqo

PSIQUIS – higher mind

POQPO - Luminous energy sphere or Aura

QANCHIS PATA NAN – ladder of the 7 rungs of consciousness

Q'OYLLURIT'L - a spiritual sanctuary

QHAWAQ – ability to see invisible world by discerning shapes of the luminous beings

QUANTUMS - transmissions of energy

SAMI - The Light Energy from Pachamama; Spiritual Substance

SAMINCHAKUY (Cleansing) – Mother provides material and spiritual sustenance SAMI through practice of Reciprocity AYNI and is one of 1st practices a Paqo learns; Sami energy flows from above, from Huiracocha or any other High Fountain of Sami through you to the Mother Pachamama and SAIWACHAKUY (Empowering Aura) the Sami is asked to Pachamama and taken from her and headed to above to Father Huiracocha and you are the connecting link. These 2 practices are cleansing energy practice & empowering energy practice. (Usually discussed one on one.)

SIKI NAWI - lower Spine

SONQO - the Spiritual Heart

SUN, MOON, WIND, WATER, EARTH - represent Spiritual Beings of the Invisible/Metaphysical World

TAYTA INTI - Father Sun

TAYTA WAYRA - Father Wind

TAYTACHA - Father God; Universal or Sacred Father; JESUS

TEQSE - the most fundamental/Universal; fundamental energies of the cosmic realm

TEQSE APUKUNA - 7 Universal Highly evolved Spiritual Beings of the Andes; Kuna is plural; 2) the Highest universal Spiritual Beings not exclusively to the Mountains.

TEQSE PAQO - Universal Priest / Priestess of the Andean tradition

TRATAKUM – no feeling or sensation; dissociation

TUKUYMUNAYNIOQ - the karpay of munay (Initiation of Love)

UJU PACHA – Andean underworld

WACHUMA or Hierba de San Pedro – Saint Peter Cactus

WANKA - Ancient temple of healing

WASI – House or Temple of Human Being

WIRACOCHA - God the Father

YAHOUI - the unconscious

YANANTIN - the complement of differences among opposites; duality in harmony

EXERCISES

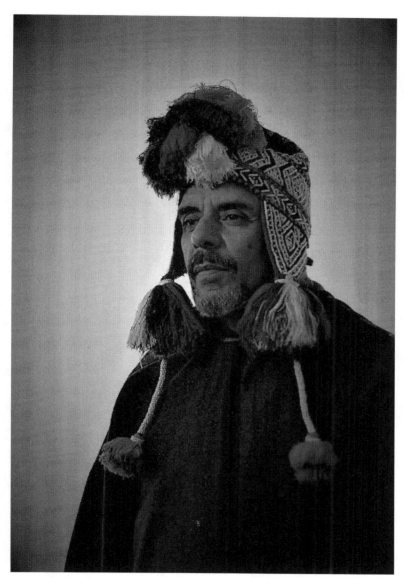

Dr. Rod Fuentes vested in sacred garments
of the Andean priests of the Andes.

For more information, on the content of this book, training and seminars on the Andean tradition -as taught in the book- in the USA visit our web site

www.andesquantumjump.com

You may send us a message to:

rodfuentes @andesquantumjump.com

Or follow us in our social media

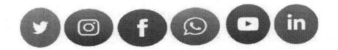

Dr. Rod Fuentes

"Andes Quantum Jump Institute"

5865 Ridgeway Center Parkway, Suite 300, Memphis, TN. 38120.

Made in United States
Orlando, FL
09 January 2023